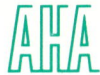

Management Issues for Rural Hospitals

Edited by Sandra L. Weiss, Donald F. Phillips,
and James G. Schuman
for the Section for Small or Rural Hospitals
of the American Hospital Association

Management Issues for Rural Hospitals

Edited by Sandra L. Weiss, Donald F. Phillips, and James G. Schuman
for the Section for Small or Rural Hospitals
of the American Hospital Association

American Hospital Publishing, Inc.,
a wholly owned subsidiary
of the American Hospital Association

Library of Congress Cataloging-in-Publication Data

Main entry under title:

Management issues for rural hospitals.

"Catalog no. 184130"—T.p. verso.
Bibliography: p.
1. Hospitals, Rural—Administration. I. Weiss, Sandra L. II. Phillips, Donald F. III. Schuman, James G. IV. American Hospital Association. Section for Small or Rural Hospitals. [DNLM: 1. Hospitals, Community—organization & administration—United States. 2. Rural Health—United States. WX 150 M266]
RA975.R87M36   1986   362.1'1   85-22893
ISBN 0-939450-72-0

Catalog no. 184130

©1986 by American Hospital Publishing, Inc., a wholly owned subsidiary of the American Hospital Association

AHA is a service mark of American Hospital Association used under license by American Hospital Publishing, Inc. All rights reserved. The reproduction or use of this work in any form or in any information storage or retrieval system is forbidden without the express, written permission of the publisher. Printed in the U.S.A.

2M-10/85-0056

Sandra L. Weiss, Editor
Peggy DuMais, Production Coordinator
Patrick J. Kane, Director, Graphic Design
Marjorie E. Weissman, Manager, Book Editorial
Dorothy Saxner, Vice-President, Books

RA
975
.R87
M36
1986

Contents

Foreword vii
    by James G. Schuman

Chapter 1. Change and the Corporate Model 1
    by Donald F. Phillips and Sandra L. Weiss

Chapter 2. Management of Change 9
    by Donald F. Phillips and Sandra L. Weiss

Chapter 3. Institutional Organization and Evaluation 19
    by Donald F. Phillips and Sandra L. Weiss

Chapter 4. Financial Management Issues 39
    by Roger C. Nauert

Chapter 5. Institutional Planning 51
    by Joseph P. Peters

Chapter 6. Marketing 65
    by Sandra L. Weiss and Donald F. Phillips

Chapter 7. Diversification: Response to Community Need 95
    by Sandra L. Weiss and Donald F. Phillips

Chapter 8. Management Options 123
    by Montague Brown and Barbara P. McCool

Chapter 9. Physician Recruitment 143
    by Joe B. Lawley and H. Neil Copelan

Bibliography 157

Figures

Figure 4-1. Net Surplus (Loss) per DRG 46

Figure 5-1. Five Basic Elements of Strategic Planning 55

Figure 6-1. Planning and Marketing Activities 73

Figure 6-2. Position of Marketing Function
for a 50-Bed to 150-Bed Hospital..................................74

Figure 6-3. Suggestions for Market Audit..78

Figure 6-4. The Marketing Audit...86

Figure 6-5. A Sample Marketing Assessment/Audit 90

Figure 9-1. Information Included on Index Card for Each Candidate...152

Tables

Table 4-1. PCU Marginal Cost Model 43
Table 4-2. Direct and Indirect Cost of DRGs 47
Table 6-1. Reasons for Rising Interest in Hospital Marketing 68
Table 6-2. Examples of Potential Hospital Markets and the Products They Purchase 71
Table 6-3. General Marketing Information 80
Table 7-1. Diversification Alternatives for Rural Hospitals 110

The Authors

American Hospital Association staff members **Sandra L. Weiss, Donald F. Phillips**, and **James G. Schuman** served as editors of and contributors to this book. In addition, the following knowledgeable authorities in the health care field who are familiar with the special needs of rural hospitals contributed various chapters to this book: **Montague Brown**, Dr.P.H., J.D., president, Strategic Management Services, Inc., Shawnee Mission, Kansas; **H. Neil Copelan**, administrator, Crisp County Hospital, Cordele, Georgia; **Joe B. Lawley**, Ph.D., assistant executive secretary, State Medical Education Board of Georgia, Atlanta, Georgia; **Barbara P. McCool**, Ph.D., executive vice-president, Strategic Management Services, Inc., Shawnee Mission, Kansas; **Roger C. Nauert**, partner, Alexander Grant & Company, Chicago; and **Joseph P. Peters**, F.A.C.H.A., consultant, Philadelphia.

Foreword

As a person who was raised in rural America, who has worked as the chief executive officer of a 31-bed hospital and a 32-bed nursing home, and whose parents and grandparents live in rural areas, I have great respect for the value of rural hospitals and the care they provide to rural Americans. Rural hospitals are the entry point to the health care system for millions of Americans. Without these hospitals, access to health care delivery in much of rural America may be literally hundreds of miles away.

The health care delivery system as we know it today is changing drastically, and rural hospitals need to be aware of these changes and open to new alternatives. This book discusses these changes and provides ideas on how to organize for and manage the changes that are taking place. In addition, it identifies opportunities for diversification, presents approaches for planning and marketing, and provides information on management options for small or rural hospitals.

This book could not have been published without the guidance, leadership, and forethought of Shirley Ann Munroe. During her more than 20 years of service as the chief executive officer of a 43-bed hospital in northern California, she became a leader of and a spokesperson for small and rural hospitals. As the first director of the American Hospital Association's Section for Small or Rural Hospitals and now as vice-president of the American Hospital Association's Constituency Sections, she has diligently worked to make information available to the nation's small and rural hospitals. In this regard, she has served as an inspiration to me in my own efforts to develop an awareness by others of the important role that small and rural hospitals have in our health care delivery system.

James G. Schuman
Director, Section for Small or Rural Hospitals
American Hospital Association
September 1985

Chapter 1
Change and the Corporate Model

Donald F. Phillips
Sandra L. Weiss

From the 1960s to the 1970s, the key change in health care was a shift from the Great Society optimistic approach of massive expansion of government social welfare programs to the pessimistic approach of restrictive legislation. By the 1980s, all segments of society had become aware of limits on the availability of materials and energy, and throughout the remainder of the 1980s, the basic problem for hospitals will continue to be limited resources.

This shift from expansion to limitation has made reduction of the rising cost of health care a national priority. To this end, in March 1983, Congress approved a prospective fixed-price system based on diagnosis-related groups. This system not only radically alters the way hospitals are paid for Medicare services but also provides far-reaching incentives for hospitals to control costs.

For rural hospitals especially, the impact of this shift toward restrictive use of resources has been dramatic. The financial condition of rural hospitals has weakened as the economic base of rural areas has eroded and the reimbursement base for government-paid services has diminished. Also, in some areas, the manpower needs of small and rural hospitals may be critical.

How can administrators of rural hospitals manage financial, personnel, and material resources efficiently and effectively, given the prevailing demands for services and the regulations on institutional operations? This book suggests ways for managers in rural hospitals to assess the direction and extent of the internal and external forces affecting their hospitals, to determine or reaffirm the role of their institutions in providing services for the community, to obtain the resources required to provide these services, and to find the means for improving skills in managing these resources.

Chapter 1/Change and the Corporate Model

The book makes certain assumptions about management philosophy and the direction it needs to take if hospitals are to cope with the resource problems facing them. Each assumption builds on the preceding one:

- Change is inevitable and unavoidable.
- Adaptation to change is required if hospitals are to survive.
- Adaptation to change requires innovative and creative management.
- Adaptive changes must take into account the relationships between hospitals and their communities.
- A corporate model of management is the most appropriate way to implement innovative and responsible institutional management practices.

Change and Response

The 1980s can be labeled "subject to change without notice." Change is inevitable, and many of society's problems may be attributed to the increasing pace of change. Events seem to take place so rapidly that society does not always have time to adjust.

Because change itself can seldom be controlled, individuals may often try to either control the rate at which it affects them or ignore or rationalize its impact. In the past, for example, an administrator of a rural hospital may have thought that the hospital would not be affected by change because of its position as the sole hospital in the area. Another administrator of a rural hospital may have viewed the hospital as being immune to change because of its size. And yet another administrator might have resisted change by rationalizing the value of continuing various traditions and customs, thereby hoping to avoid the reality of change.

Management is involved with planning, organizing, directing, controlling, and evaluating—processes that create few problems when applied to an assembly-line operation. These same processes, however, are difficult to manage in the context of health care, given the myriad of demographic, economic, social, political, and technological factors influencing the provision of health care. Changes in any one of these areas may lead to unpredictable changes in the patterns or relationships in other areas, thus making it difficult to appropriately respond to changes.

Hospitals can no longer afford to insulate themselves from change. The increasing organizational complexity and diversity of the health care field and the continued government effort to intervene in hospital business means that if hospitals are to survive, they must *adapt* to the changes that are inevitable.

Ansoff (1981) refers to two different types of changing organizations: the myopic, change-resisting organization and the foresightful, change-seeking organization. The first has no way of anticipating change and therefore has to react and adjust "after the bomb drops." The other has a planning process that not only anticipates change in the environment but also explores and moves in the direction of changes that offer beneficial conditions.

Adaptation to change should not be passive acceptance or blind adherence to the prevailing societal demands and government regulations impinging on hospitals. Hospitals must accept an active role in affecting the process of change. No hospital can afford to view itself as isolated from social, political, economic, and technological forces. Even opposition to change can be an adaptive process. But indifference to change or stubborn refusal to acknowledge change in today's world can lead to institutional suicide.

An aggressive response to change may help dispel the problem of low self-esteem that characterizes some rural hospitals. Because rural hospitals could be viewed as lacking in resources and power and therefore as less than a vital segment of the health care system, some rural hospitals tend to act as if this were so. To change this attitude, rural hospitals must show that, in fact, they are resourceful and not without influence in the community. To establish resourcefulness, administrators must shift their institutional gears from a passive to an active position that accommodates aggressive strategies and meets, head on, the forces of change exerted on and within hospitals.

The administrator who is overwhelmed by change should not hesitate to ask for help from experts. Rural hospitals should establish close ties with other hospitals in their areas and with their state and local hospital associations. Also, some of the responsibility for adapting to change should be shared with the governing board, medical staff, and community at large. Because the future of rural hospitals is at stake, hospital leaders must be willing to go beyond the conventional and explore new approaches to emerging problems. Adaptation to change that consists of a reordering of the familiar into the unfamiliar requires creative and innovative management approaches or strategies.

Peters (1979) refers to three characteristics of innovative persons: the ability to change the approach to a problem, the ability to develop ideas that are new and relevant, and the ability to translate these ideas into desired actions. Changing the approach to a problem requires thinking about it in different ways or from different perspectives. Developing new and relevant ideas requires forsaking some old ideas, that is, departing from the existing situation if it is outmoded, inefficient, or ineffective. Translating new ideas into desired actions means taking risks by foregoing the traditional or automatic course for handling a problem and exploring what may be uncomfortable positions outside generally accepted management practices.

More and more, the survival of any hospital depends on well-established relationships between the institution and its community. A well-run and effective hospital bases its management policies on a thorough understanding of its community. A major management task is to identify what the community needs and to define the hospital's role in meeting these needs. To accomplish this task, an active and mutually supportive hospital-community linkage must be established. Also required is a degree of openness to which institutional management may not be initially accustomed. Nonetheless, the community remains the chief ally of the hospital. Local community support and cooperation in institutional control and responsibility are prerequisites for the survival of hospitals.

The Corporate Model

Hospitals can best adapt to change, develop innovative management strategies, and establish solid community relationships by adopting a corporate organizational and leadership structure similar to that of other big businesses. Many rural hospitals still reflect the vestiges of the traditional model of hospital organization, which is based on dedicated volunteerism. Rural hospitals, like most hospitals, have an altruistic and philanthropic heritage, often supported by religious orders and socially concerned citizens. This role of the hospital as a charitable institution, operating as a service for the unfortunate, lasted for centuries. However, as financing and operating services became more complex and the demands on hospitals and the medical professional increased, hospitals became focal points of scientific knowledge and technological capability.

The changing role of the administrative function has been a gauge of how hospitals have evolved. The earliest hospitals were tended by nuns, priests, ministers, and other nonmedical administrators. Later, the superintending nurse assumed management responsibilities. As the financial aspects of medical care grew more complex, the business manager became a prominent figure. Still later, when it became evident that the management of employees, buildings, and finances was crucial to the provision of medical services, the person selected as the hospital administrator had to have a multidisciplinary overview of several management areas.

According to Toomey (1983), the chief executive officer has emerged because hospitals needed someone who could assume the responsibilities and functions that parallel those of a chief executive officer in the corporate setting, someone who serves as a link between the operational and policy-making components of the corporation. Toomey likens the function of the chief executive officer to the executive branch of government and the governing board function to the legislative branch. "To function at the highest level of effectiveness, hospital governing bodies can best utilize the CEO as a full-fledged voting member of the board," Toomey states. "This change in the role of the CEO as a full partner of the board, rather than 'servant,' will strengthen the proper functioning of the board and administration as members of a team." Toomey believes that the chief executive officer must assume a more dominant role in steering the hospital according to shifts in governmental, social, and economic conditions and then communicating or translating these factors to the governing board so that it can determine appropriate policies that reflect the best interests of both the hospital and its community.

Change and the Corporate Model/Chapter 1

A corporate approach to hospital management has two broad implications. First, a thorough reorganization of the management team may be required. Responsibility for routine operational decisions becomes the primary responsibility of staff specialists in finance, law, human resources development, purchasing, and marketing. The days are past when the mission of the hospital was built around the assignment of organizational responsibility to young hospital administrators so they could learn how to be managers. Second, the hospital must accept the concept of marketing, which in the health care field means more than advertising, sales promotion, or public relations. As applied to hospitals, the concept requires focusing first on the needs of the marketplace and then developing services based on these needs and on other objective factors.

Some hospitals find it difficult to incorporate the concept of marketing, with its overtones of product lines, into the framework of health care services. They argue that health care is not a product, like a television set, that can be returned if the purchaser is not satisfied with it. Marketing as applied to the health care field, however, refers to a customer-oriented philosophy rather than the product-oriented or service-oriented philosophy used by commercial businesses.

The customer-oriented approach involves three principal markets for hospitals: patients, physicians, and providers of philanthropic support for the institution. Other hospital markets include community agencies, regulatory bodies, third-party payers, and the community.

The marketing approach can be adapted to any hospital regardless of its size, organization, and mission. A process for marketing can be in place even though the hospital does not have a vice-president for marketing. In small hospitals, the marketing function can be performed or directed by a person who has several other responsibilities.

In the future, rural hospitals will have broader missions and therefore broader markets than they have had before. Although acute care has been their primary institutional mission in the past, and may continue to be in the immediate future, other missions may become more important in terms of the numbers of persons served. For example, preventive care, community education, long-term care, and home care are hospital-sponsored programs that may have a more important and long-term effect on the health of the population.

According to Bernard J. Lachner, president and chief executive officer of Evanston Hospital Corporation, Evanston, Illinois, "We are well beyond the time when hospitals should sit and wait for a physician to join the staff, when we should let others run commercial laboratories, when we should hope people are satisfied with our product and service. We must aggressively market our hospitals. We need to know whether people are receiving satisfactory service; we need to go out and recruit physicians. To this end, marketing is useful not only to examine the question of where people go for care but also to look at our relationships with other hospitals in the area" (Applebaum, 1979). In this light, marketing is a management planning function that enables hospitals to make

Chapter 1/Change and the Corporate Model

consumers aware of their facilities and services, to help consumers understand the manner in which these facilities and resources can be used, and to give consumers an opportunity to measure what hospitals are providing.

The Medicare prospective pricing system and other changes in the delivery of hospital care services are certain to accelerate the need for hospitals to adopt a more businesslike attitude. Bernard Dickens, Sr., director, Office of Hospital Management Programs, American Hospital Association, Chicago, Illinois, has identified two major challenges for managers under Medicare prospective pricing: managing productivity (that is, the unit costs of all inputs, such as employees, supplies, equipment, energy, and overhead costs) and managing volumes (that is, the types and amount of services provided and the number and types of patients served). "Managing productivity and volumes under prospective pricing will not be a simple task," Dickens says. "It will require changes throughout the institution and close collaboration between management and the medical staff. There will be difficult decisions and conflicts along the way. Top-level commitment—emanating from the governing board and flowing through the ranks of executive management, medical staff, and middle management—is critical to meeting the challenges of prospective pricing" (Dickens, 1983). Such collaboration and commitment during the transition from retrospective cost-based reimbursement to a prospective fixed-price system can best be accomplished in a corporate-style setting in which the lines of authority and the relationships between organizational units are clearly defined.

Robert Sigmond, senior program consultant with the Robert Wood Johnson Foundation, Princeton, New Jersey, predicts that the federal government will be "throttling down" on health care providers in this era of reduced resources. According to Sigmond, instead of relying on the regulation approach to reducing health care costs, "the government will use a meat axe rather than a scalpel in making cost cuts simply because the government doesn't have the time for regulatory approaches to the problem." Sigmond believes that "the era of reduced resources for health care will give hospitals the opportunity for 'fantastic innovation.' The throttling down by the government will require hospitals to organize themselves as 'cost-effective health systems centers.'" He points out that the two previous major eras of reduced resources, namely, the Great Depression and World War II, did not lead to reduced expectations by hospitals. "Although they had a rough time during the Depression, they survived even without federal health programs. It was a period of great innovation—Blue Cross and Blue Shield got started," Sigmond said, "and, by and large, people got the health care they needed." Communities faced impossible situations with innovation rather than despair (The Times Are Changing, 1983).

Today, society expects its institutions to manage health care resources effectively and efficiently. Although hospitals will continue to be viewed as the institutional framework for health care, in the coming years they will also be faced with reduced resources and increased demands for services. To accommodate these changes, hospitals will have to expand their focus from beds and inpatient services to programs that encompass the broad health problems and needs of their communities. For many urban hospitals, change may well be in the direction of specialization because of their immediate proximity to competing institutions. For nearly all rural hospitals that are the sole centers for community health care, however, change most likely will be toward generalization and the addition of services and programs that may never have been considered before.

References

Ansoff, H. Igor. *Strategic Management.* New York City: John Wiley & Sons, 1981, p. 175.

Applebaum, A. L. Hospitals must be businesslike. *Hospitals.* 1979 Nov 1. 53(21):107.

Dickens, Bernard, Sr. Major challenges. In *Managing under Medicare Prospective Pricing.* Chicago: American Hospital Association, 1983, p. V-2.

Peters, Joseph P. Creativity in planning: prerequisite for success and survival. *Hospitals.* 1979 Dec. 16. 53(24):64.

The times are changing. *Hospitals.* 1983 July 16. 61(14):101.

Toomey, Robert E. On the difference between service and servitude. *Trustee.* 1983 May. 36(5):46.

Chapter 2

Management of Change

Donald F. Phillips
Sandra L. Weiss

All organizations, and especially hospitals, must change if they are to survive. The secret is in finding out what kind of change is appropriate for an organization and then using the most efficient and effective means of implementing change.

In summarizing the lessons learned from their study on the management of change in 10 hospitals, Peters and Tseng (1983) concluded that "the best way for an organization to manage change is the way that works best for it, the way that enables it to achieve what it wants to accomplish." The way that management chooses should include some or all of the following elements of the change process (Peters and Tseng, 1983):

- Developing an active, educated, and committed board that is able to balance the economic and social goals of the institution
- Having a committed, dynamic, and creative top-management team that is able to sell its vision and goals to others and motivate them to action
- Creating an institutional climate that encourages managers to take risks and that does not penalize them for honest failure
- Establishing a system that rewards innovation, excellence, and long-range thinking in addition to the achievement of short-term budgeting and operational goals
- Building a commitment through involvement
- Seizing every opportunity to educate key players about current and emerging organizational issues
- Using forums on resource-allocation issues to develop an organization perspective among the participants

Chapter 2/Management of Change

- Using retreats to bring up issues and increase awareness
- Establishing task forces and other ad hoc groups to move ideas into action and/or to broaden participation
- Relying on a formal planning process to encourage communication and build consensus
- Knowing when to push for change and when to wait, that is, developing an instinct for the proper pacing of action and involvement
- Knowing when internal resistance or dissension is becoming destructive and being able to pull back or remobilize efforts
- Knowing how much discomfort and uncertainty the various constituencies can tolerate and taking actions to minimize such feelings
- Knowing when a more participative management style is necessary and being willing to sacrifice management prerogatives and control to establish it

This chapter focuses on general management techniques useful to all managers in achieving the goals and objectives defined by the institution's governing board, in evaluating managerial performance, and in managing the change process.

Managing the Planning Process

Management by objectives (MBO) is generally accepted as a pragmatic and effective management approach. The central idea of MBO is that the best way to manage an organization is to get employees to set objectives and then direct needed resources toward meeting those objectives in an organized fashion. In overseeing the planning process, whether at the institutional or departmental level, managers must make sure that the goals and objectives decided upon are eventually expressed in quantitative and objective terms. Otherwise, the goals and objectives remain in the realm of the conceptual and are beyond effective control and evaluation. In other words, the plan objectives must be translated into managerial performance objectives.

Performance objectives work best when they are measurable. "Measurable objectives should include requirements or constraints surrounding the task to be accomplished, the actions considered necessary for achieving the task, and the dual criteria of quantity and quality. The measures must be challenging; at the same time set in reality. They also need to communicate numerical criteria for overall performance and cost" (Bennett, 1983).

In quantifying objectives, managers should not limit themselves to using data derived from the accounting system. As Sloma (1980) points out, "the purpose of the accounting system is diametrically opposed to the purpose of planning. The accounting system can only look backward. It is concerned with history. It is retrospective. The planning process, by contrast, is concerned only with the future. It is prospective."

A useful means of quantifying plans is management-by-exception reporting, which provides managers with a means of determining how much performance varies from a satisfactory level as well as the direction of the variance. As Sloma (1980) states, "You maximize use of your time and your organization's time by focusing only on those items which show significant (however that is defined for each particular objective) variance of performance from objective."

Planning implies change. Occasionally, an institutional or departmental objective may be to maintain the status quo, but in most cases planning is done to facilitate a change for the better. The management-by-exception approach as a means of quantifying plans continually changes in response to variances from established or planned levels of performance. Although objectives can be expressed as numbers, performances rarely can. Instead, performances are usually expressed as being above or below a satisfactory level.

Change in Organization

Rural hospitals should always be open to organizational change because they are buffeted by external and internal forces that affect the mix of resources available and the mission of the hospital. Change may be necessary to operate more effectively, achieve balanced growth, keep up with technological developments, and become more flexible in the face of uncertainty. In organizing or reorganizing for these reasons, the change in structure should be logical, understandable, explicit, and designed in accordance with sound principles.

Organizational change is especially difficult. Change can be inhibited by the policies and attitudes that have become part of a system of beliefs, traditions, habits, and inhibitions in the operation. That is why, paradoxically, past success in an organization makes present change much more difficult than past failure.

Every hospital fights to strike a balance between flexibility and stability. Although flexibility implies willingness to change, changes that are rapid, volatile, and unorganized do not benefit either a hospital or its patients. Any manager engaged in organizational change should recognize that it takes time to learn, understand, and use productively the work relationships associated with a position. Assignments of responsibility, therefore, need to be sufficiently stable so that individuals can get to know their work and their work relationships. On the other hand, managers should be sufficiently flexible to encourage their employees to meet unanticipated problems and to take advantage of unforeseen opportunities.

Important directional changes seldom begin from within the ranks, because such change is tantamount to an expression of dissatisfaction with the organization's leaders. However, good leaders can accomplish such change when they actively guide and explicitly direct it.

Change in Methods

Establishing credibility in the face of change is important. An administrator or manager implementing a change should therefore ask the following questions (Morgan, 1972):

- Have the changes been explained fully to everyone affected by the change?
- Are the claims being made for the change consistent?
- Have the claims been exaggerated?
- Have all the [legal and administrative] implications foreseen in the change been reported frankly and honestly?
- Have any apparent inconsistencies in the claims for the change been promptly explained?
- Have all opponents' arguments against the idea or proposal been answered?
- Has there been a willingness to discuss the idea fully?

In the final analysis, it is the credibility of the manager that persuades others that the change is beneficial. Without credibility, all the preparation and skills a manager has will not persuade everyone to accept and act on the proposal for change.

One word of caution: there is a tendency to slip back into the former way of doing things. Selling change is an ongoing process. Inertia, old habits, and complacency continually work against the acceptance of new methods. To guard against such slippage, managers should continue to monitor the change well after its initiation.

One way to facilitate change is to encourage a team approach. Managers and employees should be considered *full partners* in achieving their objectives (Bennett, 1983). One of the functions of the team effort could be the prevention of backsliding into old habits and routines.

Communication and Change

A prerequisite for smooth implementation of change is good communication. Through it, staff and employees can be helped to accept change and sometimes even to welcome it. Much has been written about communication, but it should be recognized that, aside from its narrow concern with reading, writing, listening, and speaking skills, communication is also concerned with the attitudes, psychology, and environment related to the entire range of business and personal relationships. When effective, communication helps persons and organizations attain their goals. When ineffective, it has the opposite effect.

Traditionally, communication in organizations is downward, from supervisor to employee. It is usually concerned with what the supervisor is trying to communicate; it usually implies commands being given. This tendency, according

Management of Change/Chapter 2

to Drucker (1973), is why most communication fails. Drucker contends that communication must go upward, that it must start with the recipient. "The executive should start out by finding out what subordinates want to know, are interested in, are, in other words, receptive to. . . . There can be no communication if it is perceived as going from the 'I' to the 'Thou.' Communication works only from one member of 'us' to another. Communication in organization . . . is not a *means* of organization. It is the *mode* of organization."

Despite the complex nature of communication, there are seven basic and practical prescriptions that managers can employ for effective communication in any organization (Morgan, 1972):

- Be present or informed at the onset of planning for change. For the person initiating the change, this is not a problem. However, if another manager initiated the change, communicate with that person to indicate interest and offer to help put the change across.
- In announcing a change, cover the following information:
  - Reason for the change.
  - Reasons for a particular course being followed.
  - Details of the plan for change.
  - Effects and benefits of the change.
  - Steps management is taking to minimize the adverse effect of the change on employees.
  - Unavoidable work delays, dislocations, and problems well in advance of their occurrence.
  - Need for employee support to minimize potential problems.
  - Progress in making the change and overcoming the problems encountered.
  - Appreciation for the employees whose efforts have helped in making the change and achieving the expected results.
- Employ effective communication techniques, such as:
  - Communicate more or less continuously, that is, before, during, and after the change. Provide the information in manageable bit-by-bit portions in a consistent and persistent fashion.
  - Apply equal care and thoroughness to both big and little matters.
  - Because individuals going through change are uneasy or anxious, communicate using concrete and specific rather than vague language.
  - Acknowledge risks and difficulties but put them in perspective and describe what is being done to contend with them.
  - Think about the change from the audience's viewpoint to determine what their concerns and motivations are and then communicate directly to those concerns. Remember that the listeners will have limits of knowledge and biases. Know the audience well enough to anticipate these limitations, and communicate in a style and language that they can accept and understand.

- Always keep the purpose in mind and do not wander from it when communicating with your audience.
- Edit material before it is released. Organize thoughts and statements so there is minimal likelihood that they will be misunderstood or misinterpreted.
- Maintain credibility. Do not exaggerate or make "mountains out of molehills."
- Follow up on promises as quickly as possible. Avoid making commitments unless they can be kept. If a promise cannot be made, explain why and tell what will be done under the altered circumstances.
- Use all forms of communication, written and oral, formal and informal. Do not underestimate the value of informal oral communication to gain insight and to convey assurances.
- Encourage good communication practices in all of the members of the management team.
- Strive for continuous and meaningful feedback during all phases of change. Feedback is the means by which management keeps score on its communications with those affected by change. It gives management answers on whether the changes are moving too fast or slow and whether resources are being overcommitted or undercommitted. Use feedback to monitor and revise activities as needed.
- Have contingency plans in case of emergencies. The chance of the unexpected happening is remote if the above guidelines are followed. Nonetheless, in anticipating an emergency, realize that some staff members may not be able to cope with sudden and dramatic episodes.

Communication is also accomplished by example. Management's actions should support what it communicates verbally and in writing on standards of performance, effective functioning, and innovation (Rowland and Rowland, 1980).

Managing the Control of Operations

Once changes have been implemented and become established as normal operating procedures, the manager must direct the operations and maintain the normal day-to-day course of activities. A set of controls must be in place to enable the manager to function as a control agent.

Managers should keep in mind the following 10 criteria for evaluating the effectiveness of a management control system and rate themselves (on a scale of 1 to 5) to see how well they are doing (Sloma, 1980):

- *Are the controls simple?* Controls should not be more elaborate than necessary to first detect and then correct significant deviations from plans. A good guide for control design is to see if significant deviations crop up.

- *Are the controls positive?* Controls are used, not so much to prevent things from happening, but to ensure that the right things happen at the right time. The purpose of management controls is to obtain results.
- *Are the controls decisive?* Merely setting up a control is no guarantee that it will work. The end point of control is not detection, but rather the elimination of a performance fault.
- *Are the controls compatible with the plans?* A plan that lacks controls is not likely to succeed.
- *Is responsibility for execution combined with control?* A person who is responsible for getting a job done should also be granted sufficient authority to exercise the necessary controls.
- *Are the controls focused on variance?* When a variance from standard occurs, then controls are fairly easy to determine and apply. Primary attention here should be on the definition and the detection of variances.
- *Are the controls concentrated at key points?* It usually is not possible to exert control along the entire hospital chain of events and procedures, and so control should be established at points where changes may occur.
- *Are the controls located advantageously?* Controls should not strain any organizational relationship, for they are most effective when they and the organization are compatible.
- *Do the controls have sufficient time spans to remain effective?* Controls should be in place and operational throughout the period planned.
- *Are the controls in the hands of qualified personnel?* Only managers who are qualified to use controls should be given control, but controls should match the capabilities and expected performance of the managers who use them.

Evaluating Management

Physicians perform their duties of patient management by looking for signs and symptoms that warn of impending disease. Likewise, managers have sets of signals or alerting mechanisms that can be employed to indicate that something is "not quite right" in the management process or that something has been overlooked for too long. Chief executive officers can perform the duties of management by looking for signs and symptoms that enable them to foresee, forestall, or eliminate problems or to improve management effectiveness.

Before any dramatic changes are made in the management style of an organization, there has to be an attempt to gain a current in-depth understanding of management behavior. The following checklist can be used to evaluate managers' performance (Sloma, 1980):

- Do managers spend a lot of time solving problems rather than preventing them in the first place?

Chapter 2/Management of Change

- Do the top managers properly delegate authority to avoid making decisions that should be made by their subordinates?
- Are managers primarily guided by the hospital's mission and patient care needs rather than by theoretical concepts or proprietary interests?
- Do managers attend to problems with a strong sense of urgency and an understanding of their responsibility, or is there a tendency to shift the problem to someone else?
- Do all managers know what to do as well as how to do it, and do they act accordingly?
- Do managers and their subordinates have a clear sense of their work priorities so that they spend the major portion of their activities on those work areas of greatest importance to the organization?
- Can management freely share views and mutually determine solutions to common problems, or are there adversary relationships or cliques that make some groups operate in secret and withhold information?
- Is there an even balance between authority and individual self-discipline so that individual initiative and teamwork can both be fostered?
- Has a line of succession for management personnel been established so that the organization knows who will replace whom? Are these successors properly trained and ready to step in should a vacancy occur?
- Do managers hold regularly scheduled conferences, with preannounced agendas, as well as impromptu meetings to solve mutual problems? Do they communicate well between meetings?
- Is there an atmosphere of trust within the hospital that supports taking calculated risks? Are past mistakes discussed openly and used positively so that managers learn from them?
- Is the hospital open to new ideas and solutions, or is conformity the operative phrase?
- Has the facility ever had a systematic analysis of its performance in terms of patient care needs?
- Are institutional objectives and goals defined and written in clear statements so that everyone knows exactly where the institution is headed and what its immediate plans are?
- Are the written goals and objectives understood and accepted by all key personnel?
- Are corporate goals and objectives stated in terms of allocations of time, energy, money, and resources?
- Does each department understand how it contributes to the overall objectives of the institution?
- Have recurring questions been identified, and are standardized procedures set up for dealing with them?
- Are decisions within the institution made after carefully and quantitatively considering alternatives and risks?

Management of Change/Chapter 2

- Does the hospital provide every manager with written guidelines on standard policy and procedures?
- Are the hospital's systems and procedures documented and distributed to those who need to know and use them?
- Does the hospital have someone formally in charge of maintaining, updating, producing, and distributing all formal documents pertaining to systems and procedures?
- Does the hospital have all general policies, rules, regulations, and other pertinent information compiled in an easy-to-use manual or handbook? Have standards been established for such a manual's format, content, and scope?
- Does the institution have controls to make certain that all information is kept current and in the hands of the persons who use it? Are the materials dated for reference and review and systematically updated?
- Does the hospital provide financial statements to all managers who need them? Is the information understandable? Have all managers had sufficient training to analyze and understand the statements?
- Are the hospital's budgets prepared with the help of the managers who will be responsible for meeting the budgetary goals? Are budgets carefully constructed and approved on the basis of planned estimates from all pertinent and applicable sources (or guessed at by an extrapolation from previous performance)? Are the final budgets realistic, timely, and attainable?
- Does the hospital have a fixed ratio of managers and personnel to costs? Does this ratio reflect an adequate number of personnel, or is the hospital top-heavy or burdened with an excessive number of personnel?
- Does the hospital have in effect a systematic and objective compensation plan that clearly states the standards of performance that will be the basis for salary increases? Are the performance standards objective and measurable? Do all the hospital's employees understand the performance standards?
- Is management held accountable for performance standards?
- Is the basic operating philosophy of the institution one that treats its human resources as basically intelligent, understanding, and capable?
- Does the management team maintain a minimum of centralized control in a few required areas while at the same time delegating large amounts of authority to lower levels?
- Does the hospital try to develop its managerial team by new assignments and changing responsibilities as well as through specialized and pertinent training?
- Are the present and potential managerial forces in the hospital picked solely on the basis of their past track records as well as proven ability? Are good performers promoted quickly?
- Does the hospital add new services as soon as they become known while routinely modifying or phasing out older services? Has this been done in the last six months, the last two years, or not at all in the past five years? Is there a general stagnation in improving services?

Chapter 2/Management of Change

- Does the hospital enjoy good relations in the community? Do surveys or audits show generally positive feelings toward the hospital on the part of employees, suppliers, neighbors, professional affiliates, or even competitors?

References

Bennett, Addison C. *Productivity and the Quality of Work Life in Hospitals.* Chicago, IL: American Hospital Publishing, Inc., 1983.

Morgan, J. S. *Managing Change.* New York City: McGraw-Hill Book Co., 1972.

Peters, Joseph P., and Tseng, Simone. *Managing Strategic Change in Hospitals: Ten Success Stories.* Chicago, IL: American Hospital Publishing, Inc., 1983.

Rowland, Howard S., and Rowland, Beatrice L. *The Nursing Administration Handbook.* Rockville, MD: Aspen Systems Corporation, 1980.

Sloma, R. S. *How to Measure Management Performance.* New York City: Macmillan Publishing Co., Inc., 1980.

Chapter 3
Institutional Organization and Evaluation

Donald F. Phillips
Sandra L. Weiss

Two elements that are necessary for the effective management of resource allocations are a cohesive organization based on solid professional relationships and an overall institutional evaluation program. Organization ensures conscious and deliberate actions that acknowledge accountability, responsibility, integrity, and capability in governing and administering the hospital and in caring for patients. Evaluation ensures rational actions that take performance and resource limitations into consideration.

Given the increasing complexity and diversity of the health care field, one key to the survival of rural hospitals is an organizational alignment that clearly defines lines of authority and responsibility within the hospital as well as the areas of legal and public accountability external to the hospital. A corporate structure can provide these organizational functions without sacrificing management flexibility. One of the advantages of a corporate arrangement is that it provides clear lines of accountability. This chapter describes, from a corporate viewpoint, the managerial aspects of organizing and evaluating the governing board, the medical staff, and the chief executive officer and middle management.

Governing Board

According to Cunningham (1985), the essential functions of the hospital board are to ensure survival, set goals, make plans, organize resources, delegate authority, measure performance, and initiate change. Basically, in one way or another, their job relates to "money, management, and medicine" (Cunningham, 1985). Board members install and encourage competent operating officers; main-

Chapter 3/Institutional Organization and Evaluation

tain general institutional control by approval of major actions; check for serious misconduct; and affirm, deny, or modify policy questions put before them. The Joint Commission on Accreditation of Hospitals (1985) states that the governing body is "responsible for establishing policy, maintaining quality patient care, and providing for institutional management and planning."

In the report of the Joint Task Force on Hospital-Medical Staff Relationships convened by the American Hospital Association and the American Medical Association (1985), the governing board is described as being "responsible for the conduct of the institution as an institution, including oversight of the overall quality of care provided in the hospital and the allocation of resources." These responsibilities come from internal sources, such as the corporate charter or enabling statute, corporate bylaws, hospital policy statements, and ethical and religious directives, all of which determine the accountability of the board to its ownership. Also affecting the board's accountability are external sources relating to matters such as licensure, certificate of need, tax liability, and accreditation. The responsibilities of governing boards also include contractual arrangements with, for example, professional and nonprofessional personnel, third-party payers, and suppliers. Basically, "a fundamental institutional responsibility of the governing board is to ensure the delivery of quality, cost-effective care to patients in the hospital. This responsibility results in an ongoing dedication to the patient care mission of the hospital and to the interrelated issues of quality, availability, and accessibility of health care services" (American Hospital Association and American Medical Association, 1985).

In fulfilling its functions and responsibilities, the board makes two special contributions. The first is to act as a bellwether in pointing out community changes to which the hospital must be responsive if it is to survive. Administrators can be so enmeshed in the internal workings of their institution that they can become blind to external changes that affect the hospital. The second special contribution of the board is to strengthen and support the CEO's unique management position, which requires fulfilling the expectations of trustees and medical staff while keeping the hospital operating efficiently and effectively.

The importance of the board's responsibilities requires that today's board members be of a different ilk than in the past, when board members were chosen primarily on the basis of their fund-raising record or potential. The growing cost constraints being imposed on hospitals mean that board members today, and in the future, need budgetary, administrative, and technical know-how. "Hospitals require hard-working individuals who are willing to give substantial time and to learn what is necessary to meet the growing responsibilities of trusteeship.... It also is important that hospitals, unlike businesses, choose men and women with varied backgrounds, who are representative of the diversity of the community, and who bring a range of perspectives to the board, including different kinds of expertise" (Mott, 1984). Rural hospitals should seek a balanced cross-section of persons who are representative of the community, for example, owners or managers of small businesses; homemakers; members of the clergy; young persons; individuals from minority, racial, religious, or ethnic groups; lawyers; auxiliary leaders; philanthropists; representatives of community or consumer groups; and accountants and bankers.

A few years ago, many hospital CEOs would have preferred a rather silent, unobtrusive governing board. Recent changes affecting institutional involvement and responsibility, utilization review, and planning laws and regulations, plus the impact of the *Darling v. Charleston Community Memorial Hospital (1965)* and the *Elam v. College Park Hospital (1982)* cases, have created situations in which few CEOs want to do battle alone. At a minimum, CEOs want their governing board members to be able to play a constructive, responsive, and affirmative role for their hospital.

Orientation and Continuing Education

Whether the board takes an affirmative role, a reactive role, or a combination of the two, there is a consensus among CEOs that board members need more information than they have had in the past. Part of the CEO's responsibility during the orientation of board members and thereafter is to provide them with current resources. The Joint Commission on Accreditation of Hospitals (1985) mandates such educational activities so that "all members of the governing body understand and fulfill their responsibilities."

Board members need information that is developed specifically to help them fulfill their unique functions and responsibilities. For example, they need information to help them make policy decisions regarding allocation of resources or alternative courses of action. Accurate financial data, as interpreted by the administrator, are a basic requirement, as are data on the utilization and costs of the various services and the expressed needs of the patients and the community. Board members also need information on legal responsibilities of the board, management policies of the hospital, relationships between the hospital and the medical staff, social and economic factors underlying changes in health care delivery and financing, community planning for the allocation of health care, and current and proposed legislation affecting the delivery and financing of health care.

Board members need not suffer from lack of sufficient educational material. In fact, there is so much available that selectivity is essential. The administrator should play an important role in selecting materials that are given or suggested to board members. "Trustees should not be flooded with things to read; one cannot overemphasize the importance of choosing materials that are well written and that present a broad picture. New trustees need to acquire a well-rounded understanding of hospitals and of the issues hospitals face, including how the characteristics of hospitals influence the way in which they must be governed" (Mott, 1984).

The American Hospital Association has developed a variety of materials to help board members define their role and responsibilities to the hospital, assess the quality of care provided within their hospital, participate in long-range planning efforts, analyze financial affairs, and develop an effective community relations program (Thompson, 1979; Umbdenstock, 1981; Peters and Tseng, 1983; Webber and Peters, 1983; Umbdenstock and Hageman, 1984; Cunningham, 1985). The American Hospital Association (1977) also publishes guidelines on identifying, selecting, and orienting new board members.

Even after trustees have completed orientation programs, they still need to be continually informed about the important issues affecting the hospital. "Continuing education is just as necessary for trustees as it is for managers and physicians" (Mott, 1984). Hospitals should initiate comprehensive, informative programs that are aimed at acquainting board members with the business, professional, and public operations of their institutions. These programs should include discussions of current problems and future plans for development, reports by heads of principal departments, and presentations by representatives of medical services. Such educational programs can be held as a regular part of board meetings, as regular weekly sessions of one to three hours that are conducted in the hospital, or as full-day or weekend retreats away from the hospital. It is important that board members hear not only from the executive officers of their hospitals but also from such outsiders as legislators; lawyers; management experts; leaders in the hospital, medical, and health care fields; and board members of other hospitals. There should be ample time for questions and answers and small-group discussion.

Mott (1984) suggests that a board education committee be established. This committee would develop educational policies and organize educational programs. Trustees should be encouraged to attend conferences, institutes, and workshops for board members that are sponsored by hospital associations, private groups, and hospitals so that they can share ideas with board members from other hospitals and areas and learn that others face similar problems. "Boards should consider making it a condition of board membership that each trustee attend at least one continuing education program a year . . . [and] hospitals . . . should budget for and pay the full cost of trustee education. Sending a trustee to a conference is just as much official business as sending the CEO or medical director. Trustees of means who are uncomfortable with such a policy may wish to make a donation to their hospital to balance their expenses while on hospital business, but this should be a separate transaction." If the hospital pays the bill, those trustees who could not afford to pay their way can still be expected to attend programs. Also, it is hoped that by making attendance at one program per year mandatory, trustees who really need such programs will be forced to attend.

Performance and Evaluation

Hospital governing boards are being challenged to provide strong, informed leadership. Communities and consumers now recognize that governing boards are responsible for decisions relating to their health care needs; and third-party payers, government agencies, and hospital administrators look to governing boards for making effective decisions on the efficient use of hospital resources. In making decisions, trustees may encounter problems relating to lack of knowledge, disagreements, and attitude.

A review of board minutes can help to categorize the problems associated with certain actions (or inactions) and determine the causes for these problems (American Hospital Association, 1979):

- Problems of knowledge and information can be solved through better efforts at continuing education and improvements in providing more complete information along with guidelines on how to use or interpret it.
- Problems of disagreements occur when there is a difference of opinion about who should be making a specific decision. For example, boards may be shirking their responsibility and leaving decisions to the CEO or medical staff, or they may be overextending their responsibility and hamstringing the CEO or medical staff to the point that no decisions are made without board approval or involvement. In each case, further education and understanding of the lines of responsibility are needed.
- Problems of attitude are the most difficult to handle, for they manifest themselves in a variety of ways. It is important to understand what the basis of the problem is and to distinguish between the perceived problem and the real problem. A person may have the best interests of the hospital at heart and yet be unable to function for personal reasons (for example, senility, lack of cognitive skills, family hardships) or interpersonal reasons (for example, personality conflicts with other board members). On the other hand, there may be persons on the board who do not have the institution's best interests at heart. Such persons may have sought and achieved board membership to satisfy their need for personal recognition or stature within the community and not because of any commitment to the hospital. On occasion, board members may use their board appointments to further their own business opportunities.

How is the CEO to deal with board members who, in spite of efforts to orient and educate them, are not motivated, remain uninformed, or are just incapable of making decisions? It is usually easy to pick out these individuals. They may be conspicuous by their continued absence at board meetings. A review of the board minutes will show which board members are active, interested, and committed and which are not.

Chapter 3/Institutional Organization and Evaluation

One extreme way to handle the situation is outright dismissal or other direct efforts to oust the board member in question. Especially in small communities, such attempts could be disastrous for the hospital in terms of reputation and public relations. The stigma attached to the expulsion of a board member could have far-reaching effects on community support for the hospital.

Certainly, more tactful ways of removing unwanted board members are in order. One way is to convince the entire board of the value of having members evaluate their own individual performance as well as their collective performance as a board. At the end of the year, the board should consider the following questions (Umbdenstock and Hageman, 1984):

- Did the organization of the board contribute to the successful achievement of goals? For example, did the following items prove adequate for the tasks at hand?
  - Size of the board
  - Composition of members
  - Committee structure and assignments
  - Bylaws and procedures
  - Role descriptions for officers and trustees
  - Schedule of meetings
  - Education programs
- Did communication mechanisms with management, medical staff, the public, and others prove adequate for the board's needs?
- Did budgeting and operating plans prove to be accurate to meet the board's needs?
- How has the board contributed to the professional growth and success of the CEO?
- What changes in organization, procedures, or communications should be considered on the basis of this year's experience?

In addition to assessing the performance of the entire board, trustees should assess their individual performance by asking what they did in the previous year to (Umbdenstock and Hageman, 1984):

- Increase their knowledge of and participation in the board's organization and structure
- Heighten their awareness of important issues facing the organization and hospitals in general
- Increase their effectiveness as a representative of the hospital to its publics

Umbdenstock and Hageman (1984) suggest that, on the basis of the answers to these questions, trustees should decide whether they should remain on the board. They also suggest that "good, strong, effective trustees will be willing to contract with themselves and to set their own personal goals. Have them write down these commitments and save them for review at the beginning of next year's evaluation process." Perhaps a review of their "contract" and performance will convince those who are less than effective that they should relinquish their place on the board to someone else.

There are other appropriate ways to handle a board member who is not able to perform adequately. One method is to augment or modify the bylaws to provide for a maximum number of terms. Once the person completes this number, there is automatic retirement from the board, and the unqualified person is not reappointed. Qualified individuals, however, may be reelected or reappointed after their terms expire.

A second method is to place the board member on an advisory committee or in an advisory capacity to the board. If someone lacks competence in all but one area, that person would be assigned to a special committee of the board that concentrates on that function or area.

A third method, and the one that best serves those individuals who have given tremendous amounts of time and energy in the past as board members but who now cannot do their part, is to give them honorary board status without voting power or committee appointments. This method usually is acceptable to both parties, for it gives due recognition to past contributions.

Medical Staff

Individually, physicians practice independently in the hospital under conditions granted by the hospital's governing board. Collectively, however, the medical staff is an administrative body, and all of its authority to act is delegated to it by the governing board. In turn, the organized medical staff is responsible to the board for the performance of those delegated functions. Thus, medical staff members are granted individual rights to practice medicine and collective rights to act as an administrative body in conjunction with the CEO in carrying out the requirements of the board. The official acts of physicians acting in an administrative capacity should be covered under the hospital's insurance policy, because these acts often are not covered under physicians' individual professional liability policies (Schwegel, 1980).

The governing board and the medical staff are both accountable for the medical care provided at the hospital. This relationship, according to the Joint Task Force on Hospital-Medical Staff Relationships convened by the American Hospital Association and the American Medical Association (1985), consists of a three-step process:

- Fulfillment of the individual physician's individual professional responsibility to patients

Chapter 3/Institutional Organization and Evaluation

- Assessment of the individual physician's professional performance by his or her peers acting through the organized medical staff
- Evaluation and monitoring by the hospital governing board/administration of the efficacy and impartiality in which the organized medical staff discharges its responsibility

Functions and Responsibilities

According to the joint report issued by the American Hospital Association and the American Medical Association (1985), the primary function of the organized medical staff "typically involves the exercise of particular skills and judgments generally possessed only by a group of fully licensed physicians, such as the application of medical standards in the areas of credentialing and peer review. The discharge of this primary responsibility of the medical staff is subject to the general oversight responsibility of the governing board for the overall quality of care delivered at the institution." The task force report also lists other responsibilities and legitimate concerns that the organized medical staff may have:

- The organized medical staff performs certain staff administrative functions related to the efficient operation of the hospital. These responsibilities are generally performed subject to a duty to report to or inform the governing board/administration.
- The organized medical staff may also be involved in the equitable allocation among individual staff members of various administrative duties; the development of fair hearing procedures to provide a forum for impartial evaluation of questions concerning medical staff membership or clinical privileges; and the education of staff members about issues affecting the delivery, cost, and quality of health care.
- Although the organized medical staff does not typically function as an advocate of the individual interest of any of its particular members, it may serve as a representative of the common interests of its members regarding those actions of the governing board/administration that may adversely affect quality or cost of care or the professional prerogatives or responsibilities of the members of the medical staff.
- Because the organized medical staff is made up of licensed practitioners with many common responsibilities and concerns, the organized medical staff structure may also provide a forum for the governing board/administraton to communicate with and obtain input from members of the medical staff on matters of mutual interest — such as new services being considered or potential involvement in an alternative health care delivery system. However, potential legal problems may arise if the individual medical staff members use this information to their benefit as competitors of the hospital or as members of a competing hospital's medical staff. This underlines the principle that advancing the

financial interests of specific individual members of the medical staff is not a legitimate function of the organized medical staff.
- Finally, because of the professional relationship between medical staff members and their patients, the organized medical staff may become involved with its individual members to discharge their professional responsibility to ensure the quality of medically necessary health care services delivered to patients by conducting ongoing peer review activities that result in the enhancement of practice skills. In addition to evaluating and overseeing the delivery of health care services, the organized medical staff may be required to report on quality assurance activities to the appropriate parties.

Medical Staff Bylaws

The governing board, CEO, and medical staff must work closely together to achieve mutual respect and trust in the accountability, responsibility, integrity, and capability of the other. Sometimes, this togetherness is difficult to accomplish because of differences in opinions, objectives, and goals as well as personal failings. This situation creates a need for setting forth rules, procedures, policies, and guidelines in various documents.

The medical staff bylaws are an example of such a document. They usually include a code of conduct for physicians on the hospital's medical staff and the rules covering physicians' privileges, procedures for appointment and reappointment to the medical staff, and procedures for revocation of membership on the medical staff.

Another way of viewing the medical staff bylaws, however, is offered by Thomas C. Shields, an attorney and a former member of the Medical Staff Bylaws Advisory Committee of the Joint Commission on Accreditation of Hospitals. He believes that medical staff bylaws should be "viewed as a quality control mechanism that seeks to represent the best interest of the patients. Therefore, negotiating the bylaws is of vital interest to both the governing board and the medical staff because...members of both bodies are now held accountable for the adequacy of patient care" (Schwegel, 1980).

Procedures need to be established that allow the hospital's governing board to delegate appropriate authority for quality control to the medical staff, and the medical staff is accountable to the governing board for the conduct of its members. Shields suggests that reorganization of the hospital into a corporate-style hierarchical structure is one way to achieve this accountability (Schwegel, 1980).

To many medical staff physicians, attempts to restructure the medical staff organization and tighten or strengthen the lines of accountability may be viewed as new restrictions on the freedom of individual practice. To overcome this attitude, it is important to remember that the issue of accountability in the bylaws should be a two-way street. Physicians should be given every assurance that their

Chapter 3/Institutional Organization and Evaluation

rights to a fair hearing will be honored unless, for example, such a hearing has been waived as a result of a contract between the physician and the hospital or unless it is affected by the status of the physician (whether the physician is a current or prospective staff member).

Agreeing to honor fair hearing rights should not be viewed as submission on the part of management. In fact, Shields points out that those hospitals that strongly adhere to these rights are likely to obtain favorable decisions at hearings and avoid litigation. Shields says that the physician should (Schwegel, 1980):

- Receive a written statement of the proposed adverse action that contains sufficient details on the reasons for the action to enable the physician to prepare a defense. The statement of reason for the action should include, for example, all relevant patient records identified by number, any additional information regarding patient treatment, relevant hospital policies and bylaws with the dates and details of violations or of failure to comply, and a notice of any pending litigation.
- Receive sufficient notice of the date of the hearing to allow preparation of a defense.
- Be given access to relevant hospital documents with, for instance, portions of a chart highlighted if the chart appears to describe an uneventful hospital admission.
- Receive and be present at a fair hearing before an impartial deciding body if the physician requests this option in writing within 10 days of notice [of the proposed adverse action].
- Be allowed to produce evidence, present witnesses, and cross-examine witnesses at the hearing.
- Be granted a decision based on "substantial evidence" produced at the hearing.
- Be given notice of his or her right to counsel (even though the courts do not grant physicians the right to counsel during a hearing if the bylaws do not, Shields recommends that an attorney be allowed at the discretion of the hearing committee).
- Be given the right to appeal to the hospital's governing body within 10 days. (The hospital also has the right to appeal.)

Physicians can seek judicial relief only after they have exhausted their hearing rights under the bylaws (unless a court judges the bylaws to be inadequate). The courts have traditionally allowed private hospitals much discretion in regard to medical staff privileges as long as the hospitals follow their own rules and procedures as outlined in the medical staff bylaws. "Under a common law notion of 'natural justice,' or more generally as a matter of contract law, courts will commonly insist upon a hospital's compliance with medical staff bylaws. And [in addition,]...provisions [of the medical staff bylaws] that are vague or ambiguous are likely to be construed favorably to the challenged physician and against the hospital" (Palmisano and Conrad, 1983).

Institutional Organization and Evaluation / Chapter 3

Therefore, one of the most important responsibilities for rural hospital administrators is to know their medical staff and corporate bylaws inside out. The biggest mistake a CEO can make with regard to medical staff problems is to not follow fair hearing provisions as stated in the medical staff bylaws.

Because hospitals must operate in a cost-containment environment, they must look carefully at the performance of their medical staffs to make sure that physicians provide treatment that is cost-effective and of high quality. The medical staff bylaws should contain appropriate grounds and procedures to deal with physicians who consistently fail to measure up to these standards. In some instances, the bylaws may have to be revised to include or strengthen such provisions.

Revising the medical staff bylaws requires that the hospital administration and the medical staff be open-minded and fair in a situation in which they are potential adversaries. Palmisano and Conrad (1983) make the following recommendations:

- Time must be allowed equally to administrators and physicians to gain experience with the DRG system before simplistic standards and procedures are prescribed. Even consistent deviation from the norms . . . may be attributable not to the physician's individual proclivities, but to the nature of cases typically treated by the physician, the particular service in which the physician operates, or even the hospital's own inability to provide support services and equipment that would expedite treatment. . . .
- Administrators and physicians should be willing and prepared to put their own houses in order. . . .
- Candor and openness should be expected and given. . . .
- No significant dispute is ever resolved without a measure of mutual compromise. . . . [The hospital's] responsibility to the community may in some instances justify tolerance of unprofitable physicians and unprofitable cases. The medical staff must be willing to recognize economic realities and, without compromising professional principles, accept some responsibility for providing medical services not only competently, but efficiently.
- Even when specific grounds for removal are specified, staff members should be accorded a "grace period" after initial observation of abuses of the system. . . . It is certainly appropriate that a physician be given a fair opportunity to comply with the new rules before being penalized for infraction.
- Because bylaw formulation and implementation are controlled in large measure by external legal considerations, the process will be aided by the retention of capable legal counsel with expertise in the field. The joint effort need hardly be adversarial, but it is nonetheless advisable that the medical staff have legal counsel separate from the hospital. A conflict of interest is at least potential for a single attorney advising both hospital administration and medical staff.

Chapter 3/Institutional Organization and Evaluation

Role in Governance and Management

Cooperation between the administration and the medical staff is a prerequisite to achieving changes in physicians' practice patterns, which, in turn, will lead to lowered use of routine or ancillary services and, it is hoped, to lower health care costs. Three trends account for greater physician involvement in the governance and management of hospitals: growing cooperation in the face of government regulation, tightening economic conditions that force medical staffs to make resource-allocation decisions, and expanding collective action in the name of individual rights.

As a result of cost-containment pressures, physicians are becoming active in solving problems and making decisions in their hospitals. In responding to the incentives of prospective pricing, physicians are taking an active part in the planning of operating and capital expenditures and in the development of cost-saving measures. However, the CEO must encourage even more participation by the medical staff in order to overcome the complacency and sense of professional autonomy that places distance between the physician and the hospital. A number of methods are worth trying. One method is to get physicians' assistance in establishing explicit goals and program priorities in the context of institutional planning, a second method is to encourage the participation of physicians in budget-making procedures, and a third method is to invite physicians to offer their opinions regarding individuals who are being interviewed for key management positions.

A participative approach to management should be begun slowly and cautiously to ensure that all the persons involved understand their responsibilities and the operating rules. Administrators must be willing to share management information with physicians and should encourage the participation of physicians in solving problems. Physicians, in turn, should understand that their job is to help in the decision-making process, but not to actually make decisions, which is the responsibility of the governing board and the administrator.

Performance

How can the quality of care rendered by the hospital's medical staff be evaluated? This question actually addresses two separate issues: the quality of medical care as measured by patient care results and the quality of the medical staff as measured by its professional performance. The former refers to outcome measures, and the latter refers to process measures.

Outcome and process measures are directly related. The review and evaluatin of medical care delivered by the medical staff can be used to help physicians improve their procedures and techniques. Such improvements are obvi-

Institutional Organization and Evaluation/Chapter 3

ously beneficial to patients. Furthermore, medical care evaluation, when carefully monitored, protects the hospital as well as the patient. A system of medical care evaluation is therefore not only a moral obligation for each hospital but it is also a requirement of many external forces, for example, hospital accreditation, state laws, federal mandates such as peer review organizations (PROs), legal responsibilities as defined by the courts, and malpractice insurance and liability controls.

The medical care evaluation must provide an orderly, thorough, carefully conducted, and relevant review of the medical care in the hospital. Therefore, choosing an effective evaluation system is an important responsibility.. The Joint Commission on Accreditation of Hospitals (1985) does not require a particular evaluation or audit system, but it does have a quality assurance standard.

An effective system for medical care evaluation includes the medical staff, the governing board, and the CEO:

- The medical staff selects the medical care evaluation system, performs the actual audit of physician performance with the help of the medical record department, and analyzes the findings.
- The governing board monitors the evaluation system to ensure that appropriate studies are made and corrective action is taken when indicated. If the corrective action entails a major change in policy or procedure, the matter is sent to the board for action. Changes in medical procedure are usually implemented immediately, and the board is informed of the changes.
- In the medical care evaluation process, the CEO provides staff support services in data gathering and in the audit itself. The CEO also coordinates quality assessment activities with various regulatory and accrediting bodies, such as the Joint Commission on Accreditation of Hospitals and the PRO.

CEO and Middle Management

The CEO and middle management provide the operational leadership for the hospital. It is the teamwork that develops between them that enables the hospital to function effectively and efficiently. Therefore, it is important for each member of the team to understand what is expected.

Functions of the CEO

The CEO is directly accountable to the governing board for the day-to-day operation and management of the hospital. Therefore, the CEO's duties, functions, and responsibilities complement those of the board. Although the board has direct-line authority over the CEO, this line can also serve to support the CEO

Chapter 3/Institutional Organization and Evaluation

when the relationship is strong. The CEO should not be expected to respond to the many changes occurring in the health care field without the opinions and advice of board members.

The CEO wears many hats and serves many functions. As a president, executive vice-president, or corporate officer, the CEO is a catalyst, a facilitator, a promoter, a communicator, an innovator of ideas, a leader of persons. The CEO has six principal areas of responsibility (American Hospital Association, 1979):

- To develop and maintain programs and services that implement board-authorized goals and policies
- To develop and, with board approval, implement an organizational and staffing plan for hospital operations
- To act as a liaison to the community and to other health care institutions
- To coordinate and facilitate appropriate interaction and communication among the various groups working at the hospital
- To develop and implement evaluation procedures for all functional areas of the hospital
- To safeguard and ensure appropriate use of hospital resources

To fulfill these responsibilities, the CEO requires various skills in order to manage the hospital in a cost-containment environment. According to the hospital and physician panelists in a study by Arthur Andersen & Co. and the American College of Hospital Administrators (1984), the CEO of the 1990s will need the following skills, listed in order of priority: strategic planning, medical staff relations, financial planning, interpersonal skills, and governing board relations. The study also suggests that "the executive of the coming decade will need skills which enable greater coordination within the facility, insightful planning for the years ahead and better relationships outside the institution.... Also, to develop maximum productivity within their institutions, CEOs must establish a positive work environment and be role models for the rest of the management team . . . CEOs must be willing to look for talent from other business sectors to apply the most current approaches and productive strategies. It is the CEO's responsibility, however, to assure that the hospital's special mission is not compromised for the sake of business strategies."

The study by Arthur Andersen & Co. and the American College of Hospital Administrators (1984) also points out that the taking of calculated risks should be a recognized part of the CEO's job and the board should therefore design appropriate controls and measures for the CEO's protection. Formal contracts and agreements are increasingly being used to define employment relationships between governing boards and CEOs of hospitals and multi-institutional systems. Many hospitals are finding that contracts are effective tools for strengthening the corporate management role of CEOs at a time when organizational effectiveness and efficiency require competent, innovative, and assertive executive leadership.

A report from the American College of Hospital Administrators (1982) notes that CEOs are exposed to significant risk, both personal and financial, as they make allocation decisions that, in an era of limits, will become increasingly controversial and engender dissatisfactions, especially on the part of physicians and other influential components of the community. Consequently, a key element in executive contracts is the provision for severance compensation. With this provision, CEOs are protected from the personal risks involved in fulfilling their responsibilities. Contracts can also benefit hospitals by (American College of Hospital Administrators, 1982):

- Providing CEOs with a degree of freedom to face politically sensitive issues involving status and power relationships, not only with medical staffs but also with the governing board
- Fostering greater objectivity in decision making by removing personal considerations as possible constraints in making critical decisions that might affect the retention or dismissal of the CEO
- Enhancing the corporate management of hospitals by serving to communicate and underscore the expectations of the governing board and by serving as a clear signal to the medical staff and other powerful community forces that the CEO has the board's full support

The diverse nature of the CEO's job requires that the CEO not be bogged down with the details of day-to-day hospital management. This is the job of middle management, and a corporate structure provides the ideal organizational climate for such delegation. Delegating authority allows CEOs to pursue their primary responsibilities of developing short-range and long-range goals for the institution; organizing resources; representing the board; implementing the planning process; and serving as a mediator and catalyst between the public, governing board, medical staff, employees, auxilians, regulatory agencies, and third-party payers.

To achieve an ideal organizational climate for managing a hospital, the CEO must set the tone or philosophy for the organization's direction and management. Within the organizational structure, the lines of authority and responsibility should be clearly defined, both among and within departments. Also, reporting relationships and employee responsibilities should be formalized in written organization charts and position descriptions.

Policy decisions should be clearly communicated to all persons who are responsible for carrying them out. Individuals are better able to carry out their duties when they are apprised of the ultimate goals. Procedures that are clear and well defined keep confusion to a minimum. It is important to remember that effective communication strengthens relationships.

Functions of Middle Management

The ideal working relationship between the CEO and middle management entails delegation of authority to responsible individuals, ongoing education of middle managers, promotion of staff development, and recognition of middle-management efforts. Middle management includes assistant administrators, department heads, and supervisors or managers of various services. Key individuals in rural hospitals are the financial officer and the nursing service administrator or vice-president for nursing. Titles, of course, vary from one hospital to another. The important point is that the organizational structure should work effectively, given the hospital's size, number of personnel, complexity of departments, and the administration's management.

Persons in middle management have five important functions:

- *Planning.* Managers should provide input into the hospital's overall long-range plan, interpret and relate this plan to subordinates, and establish a departmental plan to complement as well as fulfill the goals and objectives of the hospital's long-range plan.
- *Organizing.* Managers should organize their departments to implement the department's long-range plan. Just as the organizational structure permits top managers to delegate certain responsibilities in an orderly fashion, so should department heads delegate departmental responsibilities. A system of policies and procedures for this purpose should be devised. Policies should be thought of as being the expression of management's objectives, which, in turn, are the outgrowth of the corporate strategy developed by management and the governing body. Procedures are methods that have been designed to help middle management implement policies. Implementation requires a complete understanding of all forms and records that will be used. Established policies and procedures should be formally documented in manuals that set forth the manner in which all types of transactions are to be handled. After the organization's policies, procedures, and rulings are known and documented, productivity standards can be determined and evaluated.
- *Implementing.* Planning for the department is implemented through managerial delegation of responsibilities to staff. It may be helpful to set up a timetable of implementation dates with staff. The key is to have responsible staff members know exactly what is expected of them and in what time frame.
- *Controlling.* Managers must establish reporting mechanisms to monitor the implementation of the department's plan.
- *Evaluating.* Managers must be able to evaluate their departments to see if the goals and objectives have been met in the desired time frame. If the goals

and objectives were met, department heads must determine if the goals and objectives need to be adjusted for the future. If the goals and objectives were not met, department heads must then determine why.

Often these five functions are avoided because they are thought to be time-consuming. In many rural hospitals, department heads are often working department heads, which means that in addition to their functional responsibilities, they also have the administrative responsibilities of scheduling, writing policies and procedures, completing reporting requirements, relating to other department heads, and budgeting.

In accounting for their time, department heads must separate time spent on these administrative responsibilities from time spent on functional responsibilities. For example, a food service supervisor may also be the head cook. This person may find that he or she needs to set aside one day per week for only administrative duties, such as working with the dietitian, ordering food, monitoring performance, scheduling employees, designing staff development (in-service education) for food handling, setting up diets, and working with other department heads and physicians. To handle both the functional and administrative responsibilities, this food service supervisor will have to delegate some of the day-to-day operations to the department staff.

The lines between two aspects of a job are not as easily demarcated in rural hospitals as they are in urban settings, where titles are used to distinguish functions. Splitting time between administrative and functional responsibilities may create some difficulties in the way other staff members respond to the part-time administrator. For example, if an administrative slot in the nursing area becomes available, it is usually the best functional nurse who is asked to take the job. Almost immediately, the rest of the nursing staff may view that person as no longer working hard because nursing skills are not being used as often, or they may think of the new nurse-manager as having "defected to the other side." The result may be a loss of respect for the new nurse-manager. When such a situation arises, it is essential that the CEO completely supports the individual holding the two jobs. The CEO also needs to make every effort to convey to staff the importance of the management role being performed by one of its members.

A Team Effort

The most important virtue that the administrator and management team can develop, aside from their management skills, is a sense of respect and esteem for their employees and confidence in themselves and in their personnel. Although the hospital may have a small physical plant and bed capacity and be located in a remote setting, its leadership should not think of itself as limited in its ideas or inconsequential in its actions. Everyone should work toward developing positive attitudes despite limited resources. Being small does not mean being inadequate or ineffective. The primary responsibilities of rural hospital leadership are to anticipate and accommodate to the changes affecting hospitals and to marshal and manage the resources needed for change.

References

American College of Hospital Administrators. *Report of the Committee on Contracts for Hospital Chief Executive Officers.* Chicago: ACHA, 1982.

American Hospital Association. *Guidelines on Identification, Selection, and Orientation of New Hospital Trustees.* Chicago: AHA, 1977.

———. *Hospital Trustee Development Program.* Chicago: American Hospital Publishing, Inc., 1979.

American Hospital Association and American Medical Association. *The Report of the Joint Task Force on Hospital-Medical Staff Relationships.* Chicago: AHA, 1985.

Arthur Andersen & Co. and American College of Hospital Administrators. *Health Care in the 1990s: Trends and Strategies.* Chicago: Arthur Andersen & Co. and ACHA, 1984.

Cunningham, R. M., Jr. *Governing Hospitals: Trustees in the Competitive Environment.* Chicago: American Hospital Publishing, Inc., 1985.

Darling v. Charleston Community Memorial Hospital, 211 N.E. 2d 253 (IL 1965).

Elam v. College Park Hospital, 183 Cal. Rptr. 156 (Cal. App. 1982).

Joint Commission on Accreditation of Hospitals. *Accreditation Manual for Hospitals.* Chicago: JCAH, 1985.

Mott, Basil J. F. *Trusteeship and the Future of Community Hospitals.* Chicago: American Hospital Publishing, Inc., 1984.

Palmisano, Donald J., and Conrad, Robert J., Jr. DRGs, bylaws, and staff privileges: is confrontation inevitable. *Hospital Medical Staff.* 1983 Dec. 12(12):9-15.

Peters, Joseph P., and Tseng, Simone. *Managing Strategic Change in Hospitals: Ten Success Stories.* Chicago: American Hospital Publishing, Inc., 1983.

Schwegel, K. Hospital attorneys update medicolegal issues. *Hospital Medical Staff.* 1980 Jan. 9(1):13.

Thompson, Richard E. *Helping Hospital Trustees Understand Physicians.* Chicago: American Hospital Publishing, Inc., 1979.

Umbdenstock, Richard J. *So You're on the Hospital Board!* Chicago: American Hospital Publishing, Inc., 1981.

Umbdenstock, Richard J., and Hageman, Winifred M. *Hospital Corporate Leadership: The Board and Chief Executive Officer Relationship.* Chicago: American Hospital Publishing, Inc., 1984.

Webber, James, and Peters, Joseph P. *Strategic Thinking: New Frontier for Hospital Management.* Chicago: American Hospital Publishing, Inc., 1983.

Chapter 4
Financial Management Issues

Roger C. Nauert

Introduction: The Economic Outlook

Rural hospitals, in addition to coping with the many problems that confront hospitals in general—rising costs, reimbursement ceilings, reduced demand, and greater regulation—also face special problems of their own. Their financial outlook is reminiscent of those "bad news, good news" stories.

The Bad News

Both small size and geographic isolation produce severe problems for rural hospitals. Because these two characteristics limit practice opportunities for physicians, rural hospitals have difficulty attracting doctors and, consequently, patients. Also, because these characteristics limit the nonphysician human resources available, rural hospitals find it hard to develop the range of talent needed to manage effectively. The net result is that rural hospitals offer limited services to prospective patients and thus must contend with lowered occupancy rates as community residents opt for treatment at larger neighboring urban and suburban institutions. Even staunch supporters of a rural hospital who are generous donors of time and funds often bypass the local hospital for a larger, better-equipped facility when they or their families need hospitalization.

However, if a community does not use its hospital, the hospital will ultimately be forced to close. If specific services, such as acute care, are not used by the community, these services will be eliminated. Whether the community consciously or unconsciously bypasses a specific hospital or service, the end result will be the same—the closing of the hospital or the loss of the service, something that rural hospitals can ill afford.

Chapter 4/Financial Management Issues

The Good News

The good news is that the majority of rural hospitals fill a genuine need and can actually flourish if they carefully analyze what they do best and use up-to-date financial management techniques to identify and offer profitable lines of service that heed marketplace signals and meet community demands. By adopting strategic business planning, cost accounting, and financial planning and by adjusting to their special circumstances, rural hospitals can optimize the demand-revenue-cost relationship.

To a great extent, management strategies for rural hospitals are the result of financial equations that tie together several basic factors: human resources, capital, equipment, and potential revenues. These components must be quantified, carefully planned, and precisely synchronized in an effective plan.

Rural hospitals that recognize these needs and act accordingly will be survivors. The hospitals that fail often tend to be ones that do not plan or measure performance. In many cases, the signs of impending financial disaster have been there for some time, but the troubled hospital fails to see the signs and act upon them because it is not monitoring performance in terms of preestablished plans and goals.

The "semi-good news" for rural hospitals is that many are currently enjoying a favorable climate in the early and middle stages of prospective pricing by diagnosis-related groups (DRGs). This is largely because of the narrow range of DRGs offered, the more limited use of ancillary services, lower costs, and the efficiencies that go with frequency of service. The weighting factors inherent in the DRG program also favor those hospitals designated as sole community providers or rural referral centers. However, these factors will not be enough to save those hospitals that are unneeded or poorly managed. Inevitably, some rural hospitals will be closed or transformed into another kind of provider entity.

The Role of the Financial Manager

The challenges confronting rural hospitals demand a radically different approach to financial management. Unlike their counterpart of 10 or 20 years ago, today's health care financial managers must provide top management with more than mere facts and figures. They must become "proactive" participants in the planning process; they must offer their business judgments and considered opinions in decisions that will determine the future of the institution.

Rural hospitals must adopt management strategies that are based on the financial realities of their marketplace. Typically, rural hospitals must set out in a new direction if they are to realize their mandate of primary care and their responsibilities to the elderly. If that direction is to be toward continued viability and financial health, it is essential that a smoothly operating financial plan be developed. This is especially true in an era when basic health economics are likely to produce a large number of rural casualties. Any management strategy that rural hospitals adopt will require substantial financial input from management and the governing board.

Benefits of Fiscal Planning

Rural hospitals can help ensure their survival through strategic financial planning. A good financial planning process can:

- Negotiate and price services effectively in a volatile market
- Identify the hospital's optimum product lines
- Emphasize strengths, such as ability to deliver primary care
- Diversify into nonhospital service, for example, long-term care and ambulatory outpatient treatment
- Support joint venture and networking arrangements
- Maximize reimbursement from diverse categories of payers
- Monitor financial performance and solvency
- Improve efficiency of operation and resource utilization

For rural hospitals, strategic financial planning means developing a product line that is a precise mix of types of care that can make the maximum contribution to the hospital's operating margin. Hospitals must produce an excess of income over expenses; this is just good business. A reasonable operating margin is necessary to fund depreciation and working capital, finance the exploration of new services that will satisfy market demands and improve the hospital's ability to tap capital markets, and pay for efforts to reduce costs and increase profitability. These are just a few of the uses of a hospital's profits in an increasingly competitive era.

The first step in financial planning for rural hospitals is becoming alert to the signals from its marketplace. No longer can rural hospitals be all things to all people. Trying to do so will lead rural hospitals into head-on competition with larger institutions that possess the resources to deliver highly specialized or tertiary care more effectively. Nor is it necessary or desirable for rural hospitals to try to provide a smorgasbord of services. Under prospective pricing, for example, a small number of DRGs account for a substantial part of a rural hospital's treatment load. In the experience of clients of Alexander Grant & Company, as few as 15 DRGs may represent 75 percent of the hospital's revenue. Therefore, concentrating on these DRGs makes excellent financial sense.

Responding effectively to market signals requires a thorough analysis of the environment in which the hospital operates. Such an analysis helps identify institutional strengths and weaknesses and external opportunities and threats. For rural hospitals, the focus of environmental analysis should be the determination of their proper market niche (see chapter 6 on marketing). Because rural hospitals are limited by size and location, they must focus on a relatively small number of product lines that they can deliver efficiently and profitably. The key to hospitals' finding their market niche is to learn as much as possible about:

- Economic, demographic, and epidemiological profiles of the target patient population
- Patient origin data for surrounding health care institutions
- Consumer tendencies and attitudes

Analysis of this information provides rural hospitals with information about the needs and preferences of their constituencies. In order to determine which lines of business to pursue, hospitals must thoroughly understand exactly what they expend to provide each service. A detailed cost analysis is the *best* way to obtain this information.

Cost versus Charges

Traditionally, hospitals have relied on charges as a measure of utilization of the services they provide. In fact, charges can be a quite accurate measure of utilization, especially within a single department. Most hospitals tend to weight charges so that they are an accurate reflection of the relative complexity of a given service. For example, if one X ray takes longer to perform than another, the hospital will charge more for the one that consumes more time.

Charges can still serve as a reasonably accurate statistical measure of service provided, or, to put it another way, of resources consumed by rural hospitals. Detailed costing can be expensive, and the operations of typical small rural hospitals do not warrant such a level of expense. On the other hand, cost analysis is the most accurate method of determining exactly what the hospital is expending to produce a given amount of revenue.

Fortunately, the microcomputer and packaged software have brought cost analysis within reach of even the smallest institutions. There are now available a number of microcomputer programs that can quickly perform the tedious, time-consuming work of assigning cost components to various kinds of treatment (for example, an appendectomy). These developments are especially important considerations in this era of payment according to DRGs because they enable institutions to know for sure which DRGs provide a positive return on the investment of resources and which do not.

Types of Costs

Cost analysis must begin with a thorough understanding of all elements of cost and how they interact. For purposes of analysis, costs may be classified as direct or indirect. *Direct* costs are expenditures incurred in providing service and may be assigned or allocated to a revenue-producing department, such as radiology. *Indirect* costs, on the other hand, are overhead costs assigned to nonrevenue-producing departments, such as accounting or housekeeping.

Both direct and indirect costs have fixed and variable components. *Fixed* costs are expenditures that do not vary, regardless of how much service is provided. These costs, such as depreciation of plant and equipment, are incurred even if there is only one patient or none. *Variable* costs, by contrast, are those that increase or decrease in proportion to the volume of service or the patient load. For example, when service volume increases to a certain level, it may become necessary to hire an additional laboratory technician. Conversely, when occupancy or demand for service declines, staff may be reduced, thereby lowering some costs.

Marginal analysis compares the extra cost of producing one more unit of service to the revenue derived. It requires revenues and costs to be measured in comparable units, such as per diem rates and expenses for nursing hours, meals served, or pounds of laundry. Table 4-1, below, shows how fixed and variable costs can be related in the output of a hypothetical patient care unit (PCU). As the table indicates, fixed costs remain the same even when the number of units increases. Variable costs, on the other hand, increase as the number of units increases. However, the increase in variable costs is not directly proportional to the increase in the number of units. For example, variable costs increase by $6.00 when the number of units increases from one to two, but these costs only increase by $1.00 when the number of units is increased from four to five.

Table 4-1. PCU Marginal Cost Model

Total Units	Fixed Cost	Variable Cost	Total Cost	Marginal Cost	Average Fixed Cost	Average Variable Cost	Average Total Cost
1	$5.00	$10.00	$15.00	$10.00	$5.00	$10.00	$15.00
2	5.00	16.00	21.00	6.00	2.50	8.00	10.50
3	5.00	20.00	25.00	4.00	1.67	6.67	8.34
4	5.00	22.00	27.00	2.00	1.25	5.50	6.75
5	5.00	23.00	28.00	1.00	1.00	4.60	5.60
6	5.00	30.00	35.00	7.00	.83	5.00	5.83
7	5.00	38.00	43.00	8.00	.71	5.43	6.14
8	5.00	47.00	52.00	9.00	.63	5.88	6.51
9	5.00	57.00	62.00	10.00	.56	6.33	6.89
10	5.00	68.00	73.00	11.00	.50	6.80	7.30

Source: Alexander Grant & Company.

Chapter 4/Financial Management Issues

The difference in variable costs incurred to provide each additional unit is the *marginal cost,* or the additional money the hospital must expend to handle a larger patient load or volume of service. In this case, the minimum marginal cost is five PCUs. Beyond that point, all costs continue to rise except average fixed costs. The implication is that beyond the optimal level, delivery of services becomes inefficient because of disproportionately higher cost.

The table also calculates the average fixed cost, average variable cost, and average total cost. These costs are arrived at by dividing all costs of providing a given number of units of service or specific volume of service by the number of units. Because this information shows exactly what it costs to provide a single unit of service, it is invaluable in determining, for example, just how profitable an individual DRG is.

Using Cost Analysis

Historically, hospitals have been unable to determine with complete certainty exactly what it costs to treat a given patient. As a result, hospital management never knew for sure what return, if any, was being realized on the provision of care to the individual patient. This knowledge was not critical in the past because a significant portion of third-party reimbursement was based on the cost of treating a class of patients, such as Medicare program beneficiaries. Thus, there was no incentive for hospitals to know if they were breaking even or making a positive contribution to their operating margin. The advent of payment by DRGs has changed all that. In the past, hospitals dealt with any shortfall that might result from treating one patient or providing one kind of service by "marking up" other services to cover the loss. Obviously, payment by DRG, especially when it is universally applied by all payers, makes such cross-subsidization impossible.

Detailed cost analysis, with a corresponding understanding of exactly how costs behave according to a wide variety of variables, can be the ticket to a brighter economic future for rural hospitals. Although more and more of the circumstances in which rural hospitals must operate are beyond their control, costs remain controllable to a significant extent. By monitoring costs carefully, financial managers can produce management information that will trigger management and physician concern in time to effect positive changes. Thus, cost analysis can make the hospital more competitive by improving its cost-price ratios.

Cost analysis also helps the hospital retain some control over the pricing of its services. Capitation and prepaid health care, as well as the growing oversupply of professional and institutional providers of health care, are rapidly eliminating the open-market pricing situation that hospitals once enjoyed.

More and more discounts are being requested or even demanded. Health maintenance organizations (HMOs) and preferred provider organizations (PPOs) expect to barter and negotiate when pricing services. However, the cost of providing service in rural hospitals may be lower than the costs in other hospitals in the area, and so in effect, the costs in rural hospitals are already discounted. Rural hospitals need to be aggressive in negotiating discounts. In these situations, the best weapon rural hospitals have is a solid understanding of the costs of providing services so that they can be competitive without incurring financial loss.

Financial Modeling

Cost analysis is a vital part of another key tool now available to rural hospital management. Armed with a microcomputer and cost data, the rural hospital financial manager can analyze voluminous, interrelated data and summarize financial results of operations according to whatever variable is relevant. For example, cause-effect relationships can be measured in terms of costs or charges by payer, by DRG, by physician, and by department, to name just a few of the possible variables. In this manner, even financial officers in small institutions can play the sophisticated "what-if" financial modeling games that are the heart of strategic business planning.

Such financial modeling is the key to identifying the relatively small roster of types of treatment or product lines that will make the best contribution to margin and optimize the hospital's financial position. Figure 4-1, next page, illustrates that it is much more profitable for a hospital to offer certain DRGs than it is to provide others (in part because of the weighting factors that were originally assigned to each DRG). Table 4-2, page 47, analyzes the direct and indirect costs inherent in providing selected DRGs.

Although hospitals may not have complete freedom to decide just what services they will provide, some selection of services is possible in most cases. Obviously, shaping the product line will only be feasible with comprehensive modeling that traces all the ramifications of any contemplated change in service or product mix.

Financial modeling can also help rural hospitals choose those nonhospital services that yield the best return. This information will be helpful to any hospital that is considering diversification (see chapter 7). Most decisions involving diversification into nontraditional kinds of services are largely financial, and the financial imperative for choosing to diversify must be clear. Microcomputer-aided financial modeling allows rural hospitals to weigh all feasibility considerations and translate them into financial results.

Formulating Goals

The analytical and modeling tools described earlier in this chapter are only the means to an end. In order to survive difficulties and avoid becoming victims of the continuing economic shakeout of the health care delivery system, rural

Chapter 4/Financial Management Issues

Figure 4-1. Net Surplus (Loss) per DRG

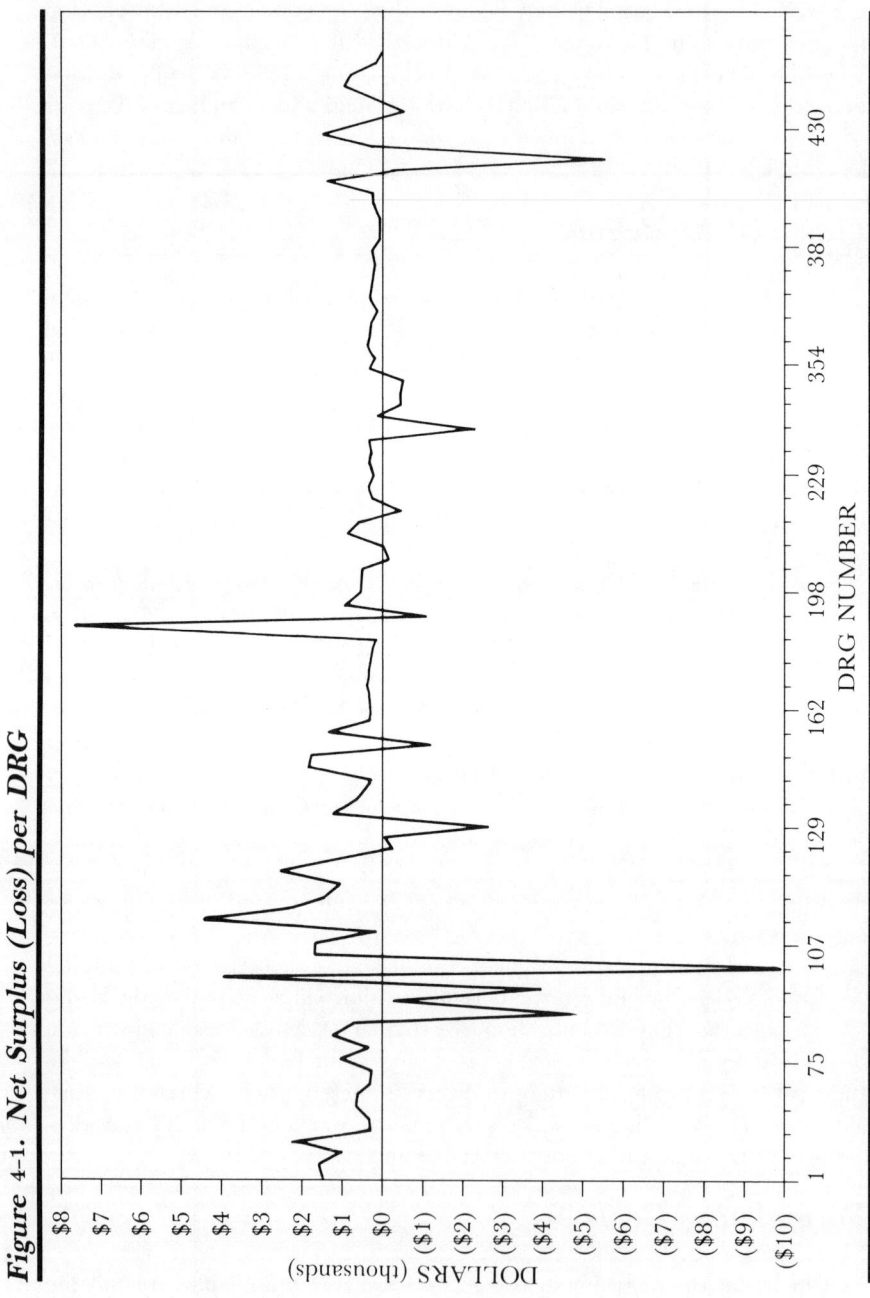

Source: Alexander Grant & Company, DRG 1,2,3!.

Table 4-2. Direct and Indirect Cost of DRGs

DRG Name	DRG No.	Units of Service DRGs	Units of Service Days	Gross Revenue	Revenue Deduction	Net Revenue	Direct Revenue Costs	Contrib To Margin	Indirect Costs	Total Cost	Net (Loss) Surplus	Net (Loss) Surplus Per DRG
Appendectomy w/o complicated principal diagnosis age <70 without complicating condition	167	65	267	323,625	31,435	292,190	113,131	179,058	119,944	233,075	59,115	909
Respiratory infections & inflammations age >= 70 and/or complicating condition	79	21	221	178,162	5,845	172,317	48,501	123,816	65,258	113,759	58,558	2,788
Simple pneumonia & pleurisy age 18-69 without complicating condition	90	32	206	691,575	65,935	625,639	255,279	370,361	266,191	521,470	104,170	3,255

Source: Alexander Grant & Company, DRG 1,2,3!.

Chapter 4/Financial Management Issues

hospitals must fashion and implement workable short-term and long-term goals. A detailed financial analysis uncovers an institution's options and permits the formulation of goals.

Goal formulation is probably the most difficult task in financial planning. The questions that must be asked in the goal-setting process are fundamental and far-reaching. A hospital's future depends on how these questions are answered. A useful approach to answering these questions and setting goals for the institution is to compare management's desires and philosophies with an analyses of the environment.

As goals are formulated and ranked, they must be supported by quantifiable measures of progress, which are known as objectives. To be useful, objectives must be measurable. By measuring the institution's progress in achieving objectives, it is possible to gain invaluable management and marketing information, which, in turn, feeds the analytical process in the future.

Goals and objectives can be stated and achieved in a variety of ways. Choosing the best path requires an understanding of not only the revenue produced by a given alternative, but also the resulting changes in service design and patient mix and the effect of the changes on financial viability.

A change in service mix can have far-reaching effects on the care provided. Health care organizations are labor-intensive enterprises. Expanding, contracting, or eliminating a service all imply a reallocation of staff, space, and other dollar-value resources that must be carefully considered before commitments are made.

Financial Management Considerations

The bottom line in financial planning must be to improve the fiscal strength of the hospital. The microcomputer has greatly enhanced the ability of even small institutions to create financial statements that make such analysis not only possible, but relatively easy.

The financial manager seeks to reduce the uncertainty inherent in any future venture by projecting the outcomes in terms of comparative financial results. This can be accomplished in the format of multiyear financial statements that show:

- Growth in net worth (the balance sheet)
- Improved income and cash flow (the income statement)
- Positive changes in financial position or fund balances
- Capacity for debt service coverage

Conclusion

Sound financial analysis that monitors performance and shapes strategic planning is a necessity for rural hospitals. On the basis of observations of the health

Financial Management Issues/Chapter 4

care industry and conversations with industry leaders, the author predicts that up to 10 percent of the hospitals in this country face closure, and a significant number of them are likely to be rural hospitals.

To avoid such a fate, rural hospitals must take the offensive by analyzing their internal and external environment and planning accordingly while there is still time. The rural hospitals that survive will be the ones that understand their operations, costs, and potential revenues and that formulate a solid financial plan to carry them through the challenges that lie ahead. Such a careful consideration of financial aspects will bring "good news" to the communities that these rural hospitals serve.

Chapter 5

Institutional Planning

Joseph P. Peters

In today's rapidly changing, uncertain environment, hospital leaders are realizing more and more that they simply cannot sit back and wait for things to happen. They are learning, painfully at times, that however successful their hospital's efforts may have been in the past, there are no guarantees that their efforts will continue to be successful in the future. Those who are still not convinced that they must prepare for change will find ample evidence in the business sections of daily newspapers of all types of commercial and industrial ventures that have been battered by change or that have gone under because of their inability to manage change to their advantage.

In recent decades, planning, that is, taking advance actions to produce a desired outcome or shape a better future, has surfaced as a key approach to managing change. In fact, planning is now widely accepted in management circles as an essential and inseparable ingredient of good management.

Planning in the sense of predicting the future and preparing for it has itself also changed. Contemporary approaches to planning focus on developing strategies to exploit new opportunities or to avert potential dangers as a first step in preparing operational short-term plans and budgets. The notion of a master plan that would chart specific actions over a five-year or longer period has been buried by the unforeseeable nature of today's economic environment.

Planning is, of course, not new to the health care scene. Hospitals and other providers of health care services have engaged in some sort of planning effort whenever they constructed new facilities, established new programs, or expanded existing services. Since the inception of the Medicare program and even earlier, planning has been increasingly promoted as an essential condition for hospital survival and change. Indeed, it was not long until the federal government, reimbursement bodies, and the Joint Commission on Accreditation of Hospitals mandated planning as a condition for participation in their respective programs. Health systems agencies, business coalitions for health, and other local health planning groups have also insisted that institutional planning be an essential underpinning in the development of local health care arrangements or in meeting the expectations and requirements of P.L. 93-641 and various state certificate-of-need programs.

All this emphasis on planning could lead to the conclusion that not only do most hospitals carry out an organized planning venture but they also do it well. Unfortunately, neither is so. Many small hospitals still cling to the notion that planning is something that can be done only by large hospitals with the necessary resources and skills to do it properly. As a result, they either drop the matter completely or turn the task over to a consultant. Even many large hospitals with highly skilled staffs and extensive service programs are so concerned with day-to-day operational matters or with crises demanding immediate attention that they do not pay much attention to the future, much less do anything about it.

Yet it is obvious that unless leaders in all types of hospitals—large and small, rural and urban, governmental, investor-owned, and voluntary—raise their sights to focus on the future by carrying out an effective planning activity, they may encounter a future that may well be distasteful to them, if indeed their institutions have any future at all. McMillan (1985) trumpets a note of warning that is best summarized in the title of his book *Planning for Survival*. He pleads with hospitals to get seriously involved in planning and adds the encouraging remark that if they do so and if they involve the right people, they can do much to shape their own destinies.

Planning is not a complicated task, although some people and some texts try to make it so. Actually, *planning is nothing more than an effort by an organization or an individual to make something new or different happen that might not otherwise happen in the absence of a plan.* Strategic planning is the aspect of planning that focuses an organization's attention on outside change and its potential impact on what the organization does or aspires to do. Strategic planning is a more sophisticated approach to dealing with change than the master plan or predict-and-prepare approaches that characterized earlier institutional planning efforts. In some ways, strategic planning is easier to carry out than these earlier approaches because it downplays the need for accurate forecasts of the future, which are, in any event, not possible in today's economic climate.

Two Approaches

There are two approaches that can be applied to any hospital strategic planning effort. The first is a way of looking at the future and learning how to deal with it. The second entails a series of questions that enable a hospital's leadership to make choices in dealing with change. Both approaches recognized the individuality of organizations and the problems they face as well as the perceptual underpinnings and value judgments that are at the bottom of all managerial decisions. Both approaches also imply that individual organizations manage change differently and that there are no quick fixes to the problems and challenges that an organization faces.

Kasten (1980) outlines the first approach to thinking strategically:

- *Here's how we see the situation* (what's happening outside and the organization's internal capabilities and limitations).
- *Here's what we believe is going to happen* (some assumptions and forecasts of future happenings).
- *Here's how we may be affected* (the implications of what may happen to the organization).
- *Here's what we intend to do about it* (some specific moves or strategies to capitalize on new or emerging opportunities, to minimize or avert obvious threats, or to resolve problems that loom in the future).
- *Here's how we intend to do it* (the development of action plans that specify what is to be done, who will do it, and other operational details).

Andrews (1980) lists four questions that can quickly enable a hospital's leadership to pinpoint future strategies:

- What *might we do* in terms of environmental and local market opportunities?
- What *can we do* in terms of organizational competence, resources, and culture?
- What do we *want to do* in terms of the hospital's mission and the personal values and aspiration of its trustees, management, and medical staff?
- What *should we do* in terms of acknowledged obligations to the hospital's community, its patients, and other affected parties or constituencies?

The remainder of this chapter focuses on developing and carrying out a strategic planning effort, with emphasis on the problems faced by rural hospitals. Although practical suggestions are offered throughout the text that follows, readers who may require more specific advice are referred to the McMillan book (1985), which is geared to trustees; the Webber and Peters book (1983), which emphasizes strategy development and the processes and decisions that underlie it; and the Peters book (1985), which describes in some detail the various steps and tasks in preparing a strategic plan.

Planning Process

In its simplest terms, strategic planning can be defined as making decisions today about the future of an organization. The underlying process is straightforward and sequential. An organization:

Chapter 5/Institutional Planning

- Scrutinizes what is happening both within and outside its walls
- Makes some assumptions and forecasts about what it believes may happen in the future
- Determines how these anticipated happenings may affect what it does or aspires to do (at times, by asking the hard question of what would happen if it continues as it is and does nothing)
- Decides on the directions in which it intends to move to seize emerging opportunities or to minimize perceived threats
- Makes some choices regarding the best moves or strategies, recognizing that a few specific strategies are usually all that it can manage to its advantage
- Shapes these strategies into an operating plan by specifying what tasks are required to flesh out and activate the strategies, who will be responsible for carrying out the tasks, what resources (facilities, dollars, and personnel) will be required to carry them out, when they will be scheduled or completed, and how the organization will know when and if these planned tasks have achieved desired outcomes

Reeves (1983) has distilled the strategic planning process into three key elements: *mission, strategy,* and *plans.* Although two other equally essential elements are implied in this listing, they are rarely specified in such typologies: *resulting actions* and *desired outcomes.* A diagram of the five elements and their linkage is depicted in figure 5-1, next page.

Mission

Mission is the starting point of strategic planning. Sooner or later, when an organization looks at itself and explores its future, it must ask some probing questions on why it exists and what it hopes to accomplish. As Drucker (1974) observed, "Nothing may seem simpler or more obvious . . . [and yet] 'What is our business?' is almost always a difficult question and the right answer is usually anything but obvious." Indeed, unless management is able to specify what its business is and what its business should be, it is really not prepared to interact effectively with its environment, and it will be unable to find a focus for its future efforts.

Most hospitals were established for a specific purpose, and this purpose usually reflected the ambitions and concerns of their founders. With the passage of time, however, these original purposes may have eroded or may be only half remembered by long-time employees or board members; or else changing times, new demands, medical breakthroughs, and technological advances have generated new concerns and new programs that have been grafted onto the institution's original mission. In time, it is not uncommon to find that no one within the organization really has a clear notion of why the organization exists and what it hopes to accomplish, except perhaps in the vaguest terms. As a result, there

Institutional Planning/Chapter 5

Figure 5-1. *The Five Basic Elements of Strategic Planning*

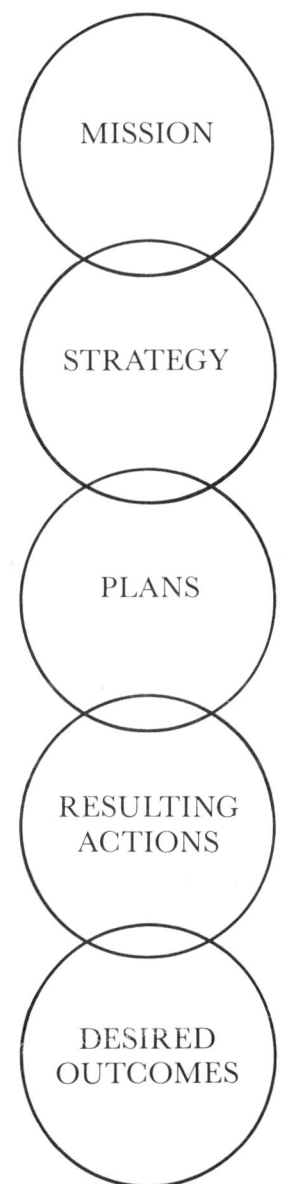

Reprinted, with permission, from *A Strategic Planning Process for Hospitals,* by Joseph P. Peters, © by American Hospital Publishing, Inc., 1985.

Chapter 5/Institutional Planning

may be nothing tangible to endow the hospital with a sense of purpose that will guide its actions.

There are at least three types of missions (sometimes blended into a single statement) that are useful as jumping-off points for developing strategies and plans in a variety of enterprises, including hospitals and other health care organizations:

- An *inspirational, highly normative ideal design* that endows everyone in the organization and all that each person does with a sense of purpose and commitment. These designs are usually very specific and highly goal-oriented. Such statements are not often prepared as yet by hospitals. (For more on ideal design, see Ackoff, Finnel, Verga, and Gharajedaghi, 1984.)
- A *broad, abstract description of role and purposes* that, in the case of hospitals, may include a specification of major functions, philosophy, levels of care, services or specialities, populations or markets served, and relationships with other health care providers. In a sense, it can be called a job description of the institution. This type of mission is quite common and is promoted in Peters (1985).
- A *list of basic beliefs, philosophies, values, and long-term goals that drive the organization*, in other words, those "motherhood" statements that Peters and Waterman (1982) observe are often capable of breathing life into an organization. Quinn (1980) says that these are what distinguishes "us" (the organization) from "them" (the competition). The missions of many church-sponsored hospitals reflect in definite language the underlying beliefs and tenets of the parent denominations. These beliefs are always the last things that these hospitals would consider altering in their attempts to meet the challenge of changing times.

Regardless of the approach used in developing a mission or its contents, a well-defined mission that challenges the organization can provide the focus for the rest of the planning process.

Peters and Waterman (1982) report that every excellent company they studied is clear on what it stands for and takes its values seriously. Many excellent hospitals also have a strong sense of missions and a supporting value system that motivates their employees to do the right things in the right way.

However, even organizations with well-defined missions soon discover that something else is needed to enable them to fulfill their aspirations and philosophies in a changing world. This something else is strategy.

Strategy

Strategy is simply a way of thinking when dealing with change. It is a framework that determines how an organization interacts with its environment. Strategy is based on the notions that an organization can make certain choices; that it can muster resources to its advantage; that it can define the market or market segments it expects to serve; that it can identify and deal with competition; that it can develop new services or products within its resource capabilities and within the existing regulatory climate to meet the needs, expectations, or demands of its desired markets; and that it can take necessary actions to survive and thrive in an environment over which it has little or no control. In short, strategy optimizes the fit between the organization and its environment.

Recent strategies adopted by two major corporations illustrate what strategy is all about. In addition to a continuing emphasis on long-time products that are noteworthy for their quality and innovative features, Westvaco Corporation is now broadening its competitive base by offering a wide range of new, valuable, and important services to its customers. Four years ago, Olin Corporation announced a five-pronged strategy to improve the quality of its earnings, capitalize on high-growth products, increase its market share for key products, introduce new products to the market, and expand its presence in certain international markets.

A hospital in Oklahoma has outlined two major thrusts for the coming year: to protect its existing market, with particular emphasis on reversing a declining census, exploring new programs, and enhancing existing programs, and to expand commitments to the care of the aged.

Obviously, none of the above strategies can be properly labeled a plan. They do not specify what actually will be done, nor do they even suggest whether the proposed moves are even accomplishable at this time. None of the these strategies could be translated into budgetary terms without some intermediate steps. In a sense, they are almost as elusive as the promises by politicians to reduce deficits without pinpointing where needed cuts will be made or how revenues will be increased. However, these statements do move the strategic planning process closer to accomplishment.

Strategic Plan

To be made operational, strategies must be translated into an operating plan that spells out in considerable detail what is to be accomplished, when, where, how, with what resources, and by whom. In short, the strategy sets the plan, and the plan supports and carries out the strategy.

As might be expected, planning is the lead element that entails the most time, work, and information and that involves the most people. There can be hundreds or even thousands of interrelated tasks and supporting details, often grounded in in-depth technical studies, and subsequent decisions that must be considered in compiling and carrying out a plan. Accordingly, much of strategic planning centers on plan preparation.

There is an easily remembered technique called the "5 Ws and the how," which is extremely helpful in translating strategies into planned tasks. Here are

Chapter 5/Institutional Planning

some questions that should be asked in sequence to accomplish this (Terry, 1970):

- *Why* must the action or task be carried out?
- *What* is required to carry out the task in terms of subtasks, equipment, facilities, resources, personnel, new policies and procedures, and financing?
- *Who* will actually do it?
- *Where* within the organization will the task be carried out?
- *When* will it take place? How and when will component subtasks be scheduled and linked?
- *How* will it be done?

Budgets are perhaps the most familiar type of plans. Not only do they specify what is to be done, pinpoint responsibilities, set time frames, and translate these into dollar terms, but they also establish a basis for performance control and evaluation. Budget plans derive from mission and strategy, as do all other types of operating plans, such as market plans, construction plans, human resource plans, and contingency plans.

There is a well-known cliche that proclaims: "Planning without action is futile, and action without planning is fatal." Like many such adages, it contains both an element of truth and an element of whimsy. Many actions do succeed without advance planning for whatever reason—call it good timing, good luck, a sixth sense, or just plain know-how. However, if the plan does not result in action, it can hardly be described as completely successful. Planning does, of course, have other benefits, such as serving as a means of encouraging communication and participation and building consensus on the need to change, but these benefits are just useful by-products. By its very nature, planning is designed, as has been noted earlier, to make something happen that might not happen in the absence of a plan.

Thus, *resulting actions as planned are a crucial element in the strategic planning process.* It is at this point where many planning efforts fail, in part because no one within the organization really knows how to make the plan happen, because some hospitals buy their plans from consultants rather than relying on those who must carry out the plan to develop it, or because the plan document is an end in itself or was compiled to meet accreditation or other outside requirements. Other plans fail because they did not make sense in the first place or because the future did not happen as forecasted or anticipated.

The entire process comes to naught if it does not produce desired outcomes. Unfortunately, outcomes are, by definition, after-the-fact objectifications. It is usually not possible to know in advance whether any intervention in the complex organizational and environmental arenas in which hospitals find themselves will produce what is desired or expected. However, this in itself is a poor reason not to take the risks that are inherent in all future-oriented actions in which there are many unknowns and uncertainties. Doing nothing can often be more dangerous than taking actions that are grounded in thoughtful planning, despite its uncertainties.

Strategic planning is scarcely a panacea to all of an organization's problems, nor does it always work as proposed. *There are no destinations: there are only steps along the way.* Strategic planning, with its emphasis on asking the right questions, imposing a notion of rationality on the process, involving the right persons at all levels within the organization, and encouraging large doses of creativity, can provide guidance and directions for an enterprise. The trick is to think in terms of the five Ws and the how and take steps to reach the elusive goal of desired outcomes, with the understanding that changes and revisions are always a possibility if events do not work out as planned.

Implications for Rural Hospitals

What are the implications for rural hospitals of the preceding discussion of strategic planning? First, as stressed earlier, no hospital—in whatever location, serving whatever market, or however generous its resources—can afford the risk of continuing business as usual, nor can it seek any solace in handwringing or pointing to outside scapegoats. Its leaders have been assigned a trust to preside over the destiny of the hospital. They face the difficult challenges of deciding which programs and services the hospital is providing and to whom; determining how these programs and services are being delivered, priced, and financed; and ensuring that necessary resources are in place or can be reasonably developed to match the organization's operating requirements. They must do all this and more, while ensuring that the hospital is prepared for change.

Obviously, none of this is easy, nor is a rural hospital's leadership exempt from these challenges. The issue is no longer whether a rural hospital should plan, but rather how it can do so in an effective manner within its resource capabilities and personnel limitations. Ross (1980) outlines some of the ironies and challenges that rural hospitals face as they attempt to deal with rapid change. He notes, with good reason, that there are many constraints and needs within the rural hospital environment that affect the ability of these hospitals to plan. He is further concerned about the traditionalism and provincialism that at times shield some rural hospital trustees from new ideas, new concepts, and new methods for handling the many problems that all hospitals seem to share in today's economic climate. There are numerous examples of small hospitals serving essentially rural areas that have overcome many barriers by carrying out planning activities that were both creative and demanding. Lake Chelan Community Hospital, with 28 beds, and Long Prarie Memorial Hospital and Home, with 34 acute care and 55 skilled nursing beds, are two such hospitals (Peters and Tseng, 1983, chapters 12 and 13).

Chapter 5/Institutional Planning

Some additional words about mission. Knowing what "business" a hospital wishes to pursue is especially important today. There is much talk and action about product lines, competition, shrinking resources, joint ventures, portfolio management, and other current concepts, all of which seem to imply that hospitals are becoming more selective in the programs and services they aspire to provide. It was not too long ago that hospitals were urged to become more comprehensive. Today, hospitals are being warned that they should not attempt to "be all things to all people" and indeed that it might be wise for them to divest themselves of the services that lose money or consume resources with little expectation of growth or profitability. (For more on the subject of values in making strategic choices, see Peters and Wacker [1982] and Walch and Tseng [1984].)

Rural hospitals, particularly those that are sole hospital providers for large geographic markets, face hard choices in determining what "businesses" are appropriate to their local situations. They must continually balance what is needed by their communities with what they can reasonably be expected to provide, given the often harsh realities of limited resources, insecure financing, unbalanced case mixes (many rural hospitals, for example, have extremely high Medicare patient loads), inadequate staffing, and the attractiveness of distant competitive medical centers to private and other patients who are deemed desirable. Dealing with these issues is made considerably easier if a hospital has a clear statement of mission that reflects the values of its leadership and the expectations of its constituencies or stakeholders, who are affected by what the hospital does or aspires to do. In short, a well-defined mission enables a hospital to make difficult choices.

When, if ever, should a hospital consider changing its mission? Peters and Waterman (1982) quote Thomas Watson, Sr., who maintained that any organization must have a sound set of beliefs that drive its efforts if it is to survive and prosper. Whether these beliefs are termed the organization's mission or simply called its underlying value system, they nonetheless determine what an organization does and how it does it. Watson further held that if an organization is to meet the challenges of change, it must be prepared to change everything except the basic beliefs that drive it. Donaldson and Lorsch (1983) challenge Watson's view. They think that because these beliefs are such powerful constraints on decision making, the beliefs themselves must change if the organization is going to be able to cope with changing economic realities.

Rural hospital leaders, in particular, must grapple with this issue of the sanctity or appropriateness of mission as part of their ongoing strategic planning efforts. For example, at critical stages in a rural hospital's corporate life—such as when it is encountering great difficulty in recruiting or retaining physicians, when it is experiencing a steady drop in census, when it is witnessing an erosion of its market because of aggressive competition by neighboring hospitals or other providers, or when it is considering a replacement or major alteration of its facilities—its leadership would be wise to ask some hard questions about what the hospital does or aspires to do:

- What is being done in terms of scope and volume of services? Why is it being done? Is it being done well?
- Is the community really better off with what this hospital has to offer? Can other institutions or providers do a better job, or can they do it at a lower cost to the community?
- Should the hospital do more than it is presently doing in terms of needed community services, quality of services offered, or costs of these services?
- Should the hospital revise its mission and shift its resources to some other "business," say, for example, the sheltered care of the aged or some other less medically intensive activity?
- Should it remain independent, or should it enter into cooperative arrangements with other health service providers? If approached by a hospital system or investor-owned chain, the hospital's leaders might well ask themselves, as did the trustees of one rural hospital in Minnesota, if it really matters who owns and operates the hospital, just so long as the town has one (Peters and Tseng, 1983, chapter 12).

Church-owned or religious-oriented institutions face still other heart-rending decisions:

- Can the hospital continue to meet traditional commitments to the poor and the underserved? Where will the funds come from to support these commitments?
- If the hospital abandons these commitments, does it have any assurance that some other sector or group will meet the need?
- If the hospital loses its original purpose, is there any real need for its continuing existence under the present auspices?

Mission, basic beliefs, traditional commitments, community needs, and other notions that some persons are prone to characterize as "pie in the sky" abstractions are unquestionably the most fundamental matters with which a rural hospital's leadership must cope. Unfortunately, there are no cookbook answers to these and other basic matters. All that can be expected from any hospital's leaders is that they design a strategic planning arrangement in which these and other key issues can surface and can be discussed and dealt with. In any event, a current or revised mission statement should be submitted to the following tests:

- Is it relevant to the needs of the community or clientele served by the organization?

- Is it reasonable and achievable in terms of the present and estimated future resources available to the hospital?
- Will it be acceptable to the hospital's stakeholders, which include patients, professional staff, employees, and the community at large?
- Does it reflect the thinking and values of the board or sponsoring organization?
- Will it provide overall guidance to the institution as it moves into the future?

In summary, the basic question rural hospitals should ask is simply this: How can the hospital carry out a strategic planning venture that enables it to make the right decisions for its institution in today's economic climate so that it can meet its acknowledged obligations to society and to the market that it serves? Here, in a nutshell, is the process (outlined in this chapter) for answering this question:

- Prepare a mission statement that describes the organization: its basic "business," its underlying beliefs and values, and its future aspirations.
- Develop some strategies that will enable the organization to fulfill its mission and achieve its basic goals in a changing world.
- Translate the strategies into an operating plan and budgets that spell out specific tasks in terms of why, who, what, when, where, and how and desired results. Here the key thought is simply this: "Even the wisest strategy will come to naught unless a whole series of moves is put into effect" (Yavitz and Newman, 1982).
- Make sure that everyone knows what is required of her or him and does it as planned.
- Establish a procedure to determine if the plan is working and is accomplishing what was intended.

From this, the reader should now realize that the strategic planning process is not complicated and can even be accomplished by hospitals with limited resources. A final word of advice: Hospitals should not get discouraged if the process or the results do not follow what is outlined in this chapter. In a real sense, planning is a trial-and-error experience. Participants in the planning process gain confidence as they repeat the process over time. Even corporate giants have to learn as they go, and even they have to change what they do to keep abreast of new circumstances.

References

Ackoff, Russell L., Finnel, Elsa Verga, and Gharajedaghi, Jamshid. *A Guide to Controlling Your Corporate Future.* New York City: John Wiley & Sons, 1984.

Andrews, Kenneth R. *The Concept of Corporate Strategy.* Homewood, IL: Richard D. Irwin, Inc., 1980, p. 26.

Donaldson, Gordon, and Lorsch, Jay W. *Decision Making at the Top: The Shaping of Strategic Direction.* New York City: Basic Books, Inc., 1983, p. 109.

Drucker, Peter F. *Management: Tasks — Responsibilities — Practices.* New York City: Harper & Row, 1974, p. 77.

Kastens, Merritt L. Chicken and egg: management and planning. *Planning Review.* 1980 May. 8:10.

McMillan, Norman H. *Planning for Survival: A Handbook for Hospitals Trustees.* Chicago: American Hospital Association, 1985.

Peters, Joseph P. *A Strategic Planning Process for Hospitals.* Chicago: American Hospital Association, 1985.

Peters, Joseph P., and Tseng, Simone. *Managing Strategic Change in Hospitals: Ten Success Stories.* Chicago: American Hospital Association, 1983.

Peters, Joseph P., and Wacker, Ronald C. Reconciling ethical and marketplace values in service program design. *Trustee.* 1982 Dec. 35(12):39-43.

Peters, Thomas J., and Waterman, Robert H., Jr. *In Search of Excellence: Lessons from America's Best-Run Companies.* New York City: Harper & Row, 1982, p. 280.

Quinn, James Brian. *Strategies for Change: Logical Incrementalism.* Homewood, IL: Richard D. Irwin, Inc., 1980, p. 75.

Reeves, Philip N. *Case Studies in Health Administration.* Volume 3, *Strategic Planning for Hospitals.* Chicago: Foundation of the American College of Hospital Administrators, 1983, p.2.

Ross, David E. Planning for survival in small and rural hospitals. *Hospitals.* 1980 June 16. 54(12):65-70.

Terry, George R. *Programmed Learning Aid for Principles of Management.* Homewood, IL: Learning Systems Company, a division of Richard D. Irwin, Inc., 1970, pp. 42-43.

Walch, William E., and Tseng, Simone. Marketing: handle with care. *Trustee.* 1984 Aug. 37(8):19-21.

Webber, James B., and Peters, Joseph P. *Strategic Thinking: New Frontier for Hospital Management.* Chicago: American Hospital Association, 1983.

Yavitz, Boris, and Newman, William H. *Strategy in Action: The Execution, Politics, and Payoff of Business Planning.* New York City: Free Press, 1982, p. 113.

Chapter 6

Marketing

Sandra L. Weiss
Donald F. Phillips

All hospitals, whether large or small, urban or rural, will have to engage in marketing activities if they are to function effectively in a highly competitive environment. This chapter provides an overview of the concept of marketing as it relates to rural hospitals by examining what marketing is, the reasons hospitals should engage in marketing, the fundamentals of marketing, marketing models, and market research.

Definition of Marketing

Marketing is most easily defined by first describing what it is not. It is not gimmickry, and it is not academia. It is not public relations, and it is not advertising, although these are tools used in marketing.

What, then, is marketing, when applied to the hospital field? In *Marketing Health Care,* MacStravic (1977) says that marketing is based on an exchange relationship that exists when two things are present: "a constituency (some person, group, or organization with whom an exchange is to be accomplished) and a value (that which is exchanged, by the organization and by the constituency)." Seen in these terms, marketing is "simply a conscious, systematic approach to the planning, implementation, and evaluation of the exchange relationships of an organization."

Marketing provides the hospital with an opportunity to match its objectives and resources with the objectives and resources of its target communities. The definition of marketing by MacMillan (1981) sums up the concept succinctly:

- Find out what people want and give them more of it
- Find out what people do not want and give them less of it

Chapter 6 / Marketing

Marketing is "as much an orientation or 'way of thinking' as it is a set of tools, concepts, and principles" (Sanchez, 1984). This statement implies that marketing must be an organizationwide activity. "*All* organization members, regardless of functional area, should realize that the focus of their activity must be consumer markets, for it is these they depend on for long-run survival." Therefore, hospitals need to train staff members at all levels to be sensitive to the needs, preferences, and attitudes of all possible consumers of the hospital's services.

The importance of this concept of marketing must be stressed to all hospital employees. Employees must be made to realize that they themselves are valuable marketing tools. In all of their interactions, both inside and outside the hospital, the hospital's employees are actually marketing the hospital to patients and the community. Because they are looked upon as representatives of the hospital, employees need to be knowledgeable about the hospital and about health care issues, such as prospective pricing, diagnosis-related groups, and the effect of the economy on the community and the hospital. The hospital, therefore, has the responsibility of educating employees about its services and its plans for coping with environmental and governmental restraints. The hospital must also educate employees and members of the community on how to be more responsible health care consumers. This type of education is a valuable component of the marketing process.

"If carried out effectively, marketing should result in situations such as the following" (MacStravic, 1977):

- Health care programs are developed so as to be responsive to the needs of the populations they are intended to serve. . . .
- The relationships between the organization and its constituencies are serving the interests of all. . . .
- Health care programs are developed to serve and attract specific segments or subsets of those potentially interested. The programs are tailored to the individual segment rather than to the public at large and, as a result, are more successful. . . .
- Health care programs are developed according to the needs of potential clients rather than to the desire for prestige by the institution or the latest technological fad. . . .
- The marketing concept permeates the organization and all its affairs. Everything the organization does in some way affects actual or potential exchanges with its constituencies. . . .
- The health care organization addresses all aspects of its services in evaluating old programs or designing new ones. It considers the service itself and the perceived benefits it represents to its users. It recognizes the impact of price, including everything the potential user must go through to avail himself of that service. It incorporates promotion, the communications necessary to educate and motivate potential consitutents to make the desired exchange.

Reasons for Marketing

There are a host of reasons why interest in hospital marketing has grown rapidly in recent years. Robinson and Whittington (1980) summarize 11 reasons for rising levels of interest in health care marketing (table 6-1, next page). Public accountability, competition within the health care field, and changing consumer expectations are the general external forces at work. Marketing has become a necessity on defensive and survival grounds as a result of prospective pricing, efforts to limit and reduce the supply of beds, and pressures by review agencies to limit inpatient services. Organizations need to improve their capacity to respond to the needs and wants of consumers, personnel, and the community in general; clarify the development of long-range strategies and objectives; and more effectively allocate resources within the organization (Berkowitz and Flexner, 1978).

Rural areas will experience their own sets of unique situations that demand attention to marketing. First, increased competition in urban areas for hospital patients will create outreach systems to rural areas. Second, there will be an influx into rural communities of new physicians practicing both primary and specialized care. Third, the growing population in rural areas of previously urban-dwelling individuals will seek more discriminating and sophisticated health care services. Rural hospitals will have to rethink how they will attract new physicians and patients and what services they will offer in order to remain financially viable and community conscious.

Marketing, therefore, is an essential function for hospitals because it is founded on what McMillan (1981) calls "this bedrock":

- Hospitals are here to serve consumers' needs. The mission of the hospital within its community is to help patients get well and stay well. Consumers are a hospital's reason for existence.
- Consumers have a legitimate interest in hospitals and what goes on there. Measuring and understanding their concerns are legitimate and urgent actions.
- Consumers in total — that is, *society* — will express their concerns through legislation when either costs or concerns get high enough.
- Hospitals that do not listen well or interact effectively will probably fail or be penalized for unresponsiveness to consumer needs.
- Hospitals that can both listen and communicate effectively will thrive.

Marketing Fundamentals in Brief

Hospitals are in business — the business of making people well and keeping them that way. The product they sell is good health, and they must market that product just as commercial businesses do. The primary purchasers of the hospital's product are patients. However, for marketing purposes, there are secondary consumers:

Table 6-1. *Reasons for Rising Interest in Hospital Marketing*

Reason	Explanation
1. Rising costs	With rapid escalation of health care costs has come a search for methods and techniques to slow the rate of increase. Marketing may be useful to hospital administrators in effecting cost containment measures.
2. Rising accountability	Legislation has created mechanisms for review of health care service providers. Providers are now required to have information to support requests for additional services and to defend the allocation of resources. Marketing techniques and concepts are useful in the development of such information.
3. Trustees and directors have placed increasing emphasis on the health care consumer's needs	Administrators must demonstrate to governing boards that the health care consumer has been consulted and his or her needs considered in planning and operating the services offered.
4. Increase in proprietary health care services	There have been widely reported successes of such profit making health care services as hospital management firms, proprietary hospitals, health maintenance organizations, group practices, and emergency clinics. As a result, many hospital administrators and board members believe that hospitals must become more competitive and devote increased attention to their principal markets.
5. Underutilization viewed as waste	Marketing provides the administrator with concepts and techniques to smooth irregular demand patterns, to review consumer needs, to identify and reach target markets and to measure customer satisfaction with services offered. Thus, marketing may be useful in increasing levels of utilization without creating demand for unneeded services.
6. Duplication of services	Marketing can assist administrators to measure total demand, assess the level and quality of services offered by other health care providers, and determine which services should be offered to meet effectively the needs of the markets served by the hospitals. Thus, marketing can provide information to assist decision makers in their quest to achieve effective utilization of available financial, human, and equipment resources.

(continued)

Table 6-1 (continued)

Reason	Explanation
7. Rising sense of professionalism by staff	Increasingly nurses, pharmacists, respiratory therapists, and other staff members seek broader recognition for their contributions. Marketing, with its emphasis on exchange relationships with key publics, provides an approach to administrators faced with an increasingly complex set of staff needs and expectations.
8. Changing nature of patient/physician relationship	The patient has become a more active participant in decisions affecting his or her health care. Choices with respect to where, how, and what health care services are sought are increasingly influenced by consumer awareness and knowledge. Marketing techniques are useful in development of consumer awareness and in provision of information about alternative services.
9. Rising interest in prevention	While most consumers still seek health care on an episodic, curative crisis basis, there is a clear trend toward utilization of preventive health services. Preventive health services possess characteristics which are amenable to marketing efforts and which can reduce the overall costs of health care substantially.
10. Rising consumer dissatisfaction with health care providers	Expectation levels of health care consumers are rising. Therefore, health care providers must develop a better understanding of consumer expectations and satisfaction levels. Marketing provides the measurement techniques needed to determine patient expectations and satisfaction.
11. The hospital as a business	Many observers believe that health care possesses the elements of a business. That is, there are products and services which are offered to consumers by competitors at prices and locations which differ substantially. Also, effective public relations and promotional techniques use the same principles as are used by business firms.

Reprinted, with permission, from "Marketing as Viewed by Hospital Administrators," by Larry M. Robinson and F. Brown Whittington, in *Health Care Marketing: Issues and Trends*, edited by Phillip D. Cooper, © by Aspen Systems Corporation, 1979, pp. 40-41.

Chapter 6/Marketing

physicians, third-party payers, employers and employees, trustees, administrators, contributors, persons buying wellness services or similar services from the hospital. Marketing is accomplished by keeping the needs of *all* consumers foremost in mind.

To market themselves effectively, hospitals must get used to thinking in marketing terms. The basic elements of the marketing process are the four Ps: *product, price, promotion,* and *place (distribution):*

- *Product* — what the hospital is selling. Product can also be described as the "benefits people believe they will derive out of doing business with you, being your patient, or becoming a member of your medical staff, for example" (MacStravic, 1980). An important aspect to consider is that hospitals sell their product to someone. Table 6-2, next page, lists some hospital markets and the products they purchase. Hospitals must segment their markets and develop product lines that appeal to these market segments and that can be supplied in a cost-effective and profitable manner by the hospital. Because of prospective pricing, hospitals will need to assess the growth possibilities and profitability of the products they offer or are thinking of offering and consider these aspects of each product in terms of the hospital's mission (Seymour, 1984).
- *Price* — the cost of services, not only in money, but in time, anxiety, discomfort, pain, complexity, transportation, convenience, waiting, and so forth. "Price is the flip side of product: the financial, physical, and psychological costs to people of doing business with you" (MacStravic, 1980). Frequently, the other-than-monetary costs of service are more important to achieving patient satisfaction. Indeed, to secondary consumers, convenience of resources and commitment by top-level management may be all-important aspects in choosing to practice in a particular hospital. Under prospective pricing systems, hospitals will need to compete more on the basis of price; "they are likely to cut prices to gain volume" (Seymour, 1984).
- *Promotion* — the communication of what services the hospital provides. Once the hospital has determined what products it will offer, it must take steps to make the consumer aware of what is available. Promotion may become even more important under prospective pricing because hospitals may be providing fewer secondary products than patients have been getting and patients will be paying a larger share of what they do get (Seymour, 1984).
- *Place (distribution)* — the location and availability of services and the "hospital's place within the entire system of institutions involved in the marketing process. To distribute health care, the hospital obviously needs to work with physicians, local businesses, government, third-party payers, donors, and others. These are therefore said to comprise the *channel of distribution*" (Fine, 1984). Place includes the "understanding people have about how to go about doing business with you and the circumstances under which they can avail themselves of your product" (MacStravic 1980).

Table 6-2. **Examples of Potential Hospital Markets and the Products They Purchase**

Hospital Markets	Products They Purchase
Donors	Publicity, tax breaks
Executives	Understanding of marketing and its benefits
General public	Fixed-fee comprehensive exams, catering, housekeeping, day care, services for the elderly, educational programs
Government regulators	Conformity to rules and deadlines, supportive public opinion
Local business	Consultation in health benefits and costs, industrial health services, pre-employment physicals, health and safety education programs
National business	Research programs
Patients	Quality care, hotel services, patient representatives, VIP cards, warmth
Patients' families	Information about patient's condition, discharge planning, kindness
Physicians	Nursing services, office and lounge space, referral services, laboratory services, prestigious reputation
Press	24-hour contact, well-written releases about newsworthy, innovative activities
Schools	Health education and immunization programs, health assessments, pre-med student programs
Third-party payers	Expeditious record-keeping, cost-effective service
Trustees	Opportunity to give advice, prestige
Visitors	Courtesy, information, directional signs, parking, convenient hours
Volunteers	Recognition, visibility, companionship, opportunity for future employment

Reprinted, with permission, from "The Health Product: A Social Marketing Perspective," by Seymour H. Fine, in *Hospitals*, 58(12):67, June 1, 1984.

In developing a marketing plan, each of the four Ps must be considered. Fine (1984) also suggests that a marketing plan must also consider the hospital's goals for its marketing function and consumer research. The marketing plan will not be successful unless the hospital has developed specific and achievable goals and listed them according to priorities. Every goal cannot be of primary importance. Also, the goals for the marketing process may not be accomplished if the hospital does not find out what its consumers want and need. This leads to consumer research, which is the "most powerful and most abused item in the marketer's tool kit. All too often it is either overdone or underutilized. . . . Research should be conducted only if necessary, and then should be done carefully and completely" (Fine, 1984).

How the hospital allocates its resources to the four Ps is its marketing mix, which is the "management of the exchanges between an organization and its publics" (Seymour, 1984). "In theory, the organization that creates the optimum marketing mix will emerge as the most competitive in the marketplace" (Fine, 1984).

Organization of the Marketing Function

Most hospitals have engaged in marketing to some extent whether they realize it or not. Any hospital with a community service department, an admissions and discharge planning function, or a program of community education has performed the essence of marketing because all of these areas must be responsive to consumers. Any hospital activity that relates to the delivery of services and the communication with patient or community groups is, in fact, engaged in marketing. What separates the marketing-savvy and successful hospitals from the marketing-sorry and unsuccessful hospitals is the degree of commitment and organization that defines and supports the marketing effort.

Marketing is first and foremost a business function with business objectives, and one of these objectives should relate to or equate with more-efficient operations. For this reason, marketing should be an integral part of and in agreement with the institution's corporate planning process and objectives.

The relationship between the planning and marketing processes can be confusing. In reality, some of the functions within these two processes are shared, rather like two sides of the same coin. Tucker (1981) has set up an integrated planning and marketing model, in which he defines 10 functions: goal setting, forecasting, service definition, access, price determination, promotion, image management, regulatory process, internal project management, and feedback (figure 6-1, next page). Both institutional planning and marketing address the majority of these activities. However, the emphasis or perspective for any activity varies depending on whether a planning or marketing orientation is required. Also, several activities receive more emphasis than others in both approaches, as illustrated by the size of the horizontal bars in figure 6-1.

Like planning, marketing is not a responsibility to be relegated to a single middle-management person who is rewarded with a change in title and a pay

Figure 6-1. *Planning and Marketing Activities*

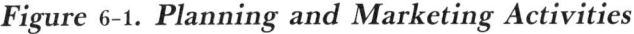

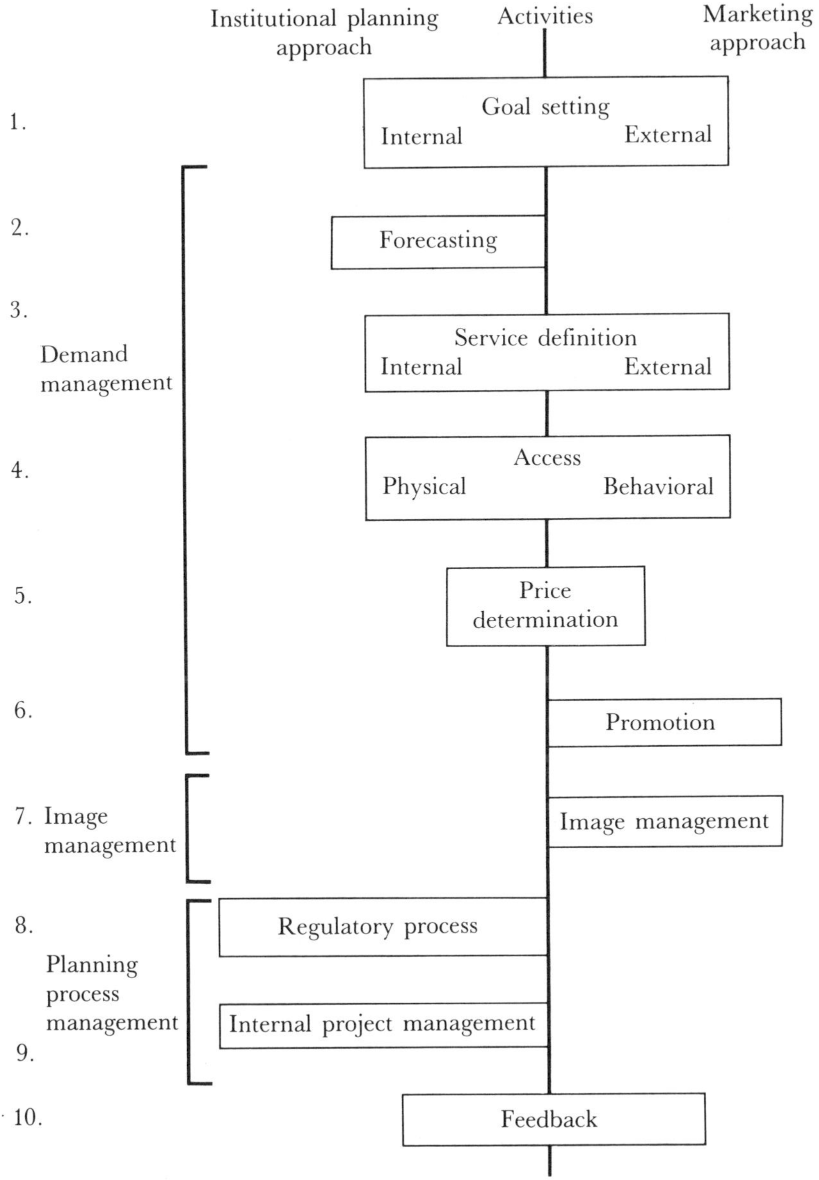

Reprinted, with permission, from "Integrating Planning and Marketing Activities in Hospitals," by Stephen L. Tucker, in *Health Care Planning & Marketing*, 1(1):2, Apr. 1981.

Chapter 6/Marketing

hike. The expectation that one person can do marketing implies that marketing is only a tool, not an integral function of the day-to-day operation of the hospital. Another ploy of the CEO who does not understand marketing is to assign the function to a task force that has no official sanction. To do so is to avoid the issues raised by the marketing process and to deny that marketing is a business management function that should be fully integrated into the hospital just as accounting, financial management, personnel management, data processing, and operations management functions were more than a decade ago.

In business, the person in charge of marketing reports to the chief executive officer and is part of the executive management team. If a hospital's marketing efforts are to be successful, it must make a similar commitment to the marketing function. The marketing executive should have direct access to the CEO or to a person at the top level of the hospital's organization chart. To be most successful, the marketing function should be elevated to at least the vice-presidential level (Sanchez, 1984). This access to the CEO indicates the commitment of the CEO and the importance that is attached to the marketing function.

For small hospitals (150 beds or fewer), Campbell (1981) suggests that a marketing committee carry out the marketing functions (figure 6-2, below). The committee could consist of key department heads, assistant administrators, representatives from the nursing and medical staffs, and a member of the governing board. The committee would be charged with analyzing marketing issues, making recommendations to the CEO, and hiring marketing research services or advertising services from outside consultants when needed.

Figure 6-2. **Position of Marketing Function for a 50-Bed to a 150-Bed Hospital**

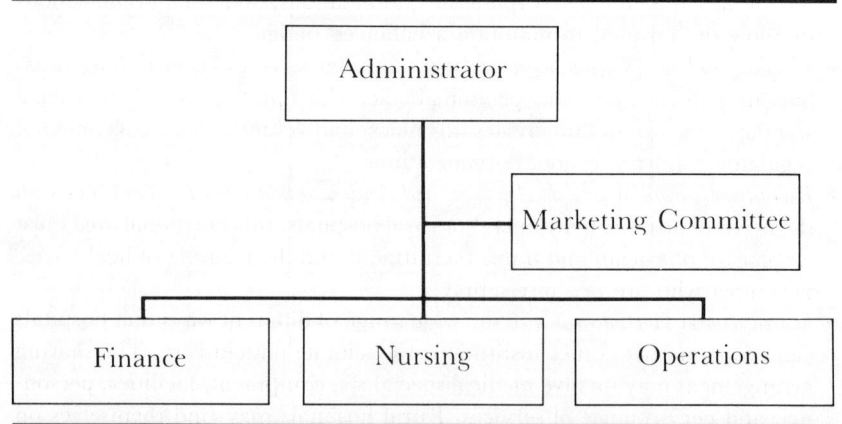

Reprinted, with permission, from "Establishing a Marketing Organization for Hospitals," by B. Campbell, in *Journal of Health Care Marketing,* 1(2):32, Spring 1981.

Steps should be taken to gain the full support and commitment of the governing board, medical staff, administrative staff, and employees for a marketing program because each of these groups plays an important role in its success. They should understand, at mimimum, the intent, goals, and objectives, as well as the methods and rationale for the marketing techniques to be used.

Marketing Functions and Models

Up to now, marketing has been spoken of in broad terms, with only passing reference to the specific activities or functions that comprise the marketing process. Although the nature and extent of marketing activities may vary from one hospital to another, the marketing framework outlined by Campbell (1981) serves as a convenient way of organizing marketing activities for review. The eight functions described by Campbell point to the diversity of groups to which marketing is directed:

- *Patient relations functions* assist patients with their nonmedical needs and represent the patient's interest during hospitalization. *Community relations functions* inform the community of programs that benefit the public. Such activities include sponsoring health fairs, first-aid seminars, screening programs, and local school career days; fostering relationships with other community organizations; and developing consumer education programs.
- *Public relations functions* enhance the public's attitude toward or image of the institution through communication tools such as internal and external publications, advertising, and media relations.
- *Development and philanthropy functions* raise contributions and funds from individuals and families, corporations, foundations, and other organizations to allow the hospital to maintain a balanced budget.
- *Planning and governmental agency relations functions* serve to foster management liaisons with local and state planning bodies, third-party payers, professional standards review and rate review agencies, and voluntary and govenmental regulatory and professional organizations.
- *Recruitment, training and development, and continuing education functions* focus on the needs of hospital personnel. For rural hospitals, this functional area must emphasize physician and nurse recruitment and the training of health care personnel who are in short supply.
- *Shared services functions* refer to the wide range of different ways that hospitals can cooperate with other institutions to facilitate patient care. The sharing arrangement may involve medical specialists, equipment, facilities, personnel, and performance of services. Rural hospitals may find themselves on the receiving end of such arrangements, but marketing can help define those assets that the hospital can offer to other health care organizations.

Chapter 6/Marketing

- *Program research and evaluation functions* are marketing tasks that Campbell believes should exist in all hospitals to review new and existing programs. This functional area serves as a resource to help the hospital determine the feasibility of new programs, buildings, or services and to evaluate the need for current services.
- *Marketing information system functions* provide the basic kinds of data needed by managers to assess current marketing conditions. Campbell refers to it as an internal data system, but the information covers a wide range of subjects in the hospital's external environment.

Confusion over the role and application of marketing stems from the lack of any all-encompassing and agreed-upon model of marketing for hospitals and the wide assortment of terms used to define or characterize marketing components. Some models define marketing according to the object of the marketing effort, for example, patient and community relations or physician recruitment. Other models stress the actual activities undertaken, for example, fund raising or advertising. Some try to accommodate the classic business marketing model, with its five areas of concern: marketing research, product identification, distribution, promotion, and pricing. Still others think of marketing in terms of the outcome, or end result, of the activities related to marketing, such as competing aggressively for physicians, diversifying into areas other than inpatient care, developing captive distribution systems, and promoting the institution's services (Goldsmith, 1980).

Beckham (1984) suggests that an industrial approach to marketing may be suitable for some hospitals. In this approach, activities are divided into two major product segments: consumer market and professional market. A third activity of equal importance is market research. The consumer market area would be concerned with advertising, public relations, promotion, and community education and training because these are activities used to reach consumers. Services that could be marketed through this area are those that can be directly selected by consumers, for example, home health care, health promotion, cosmetic surgery, and obstetrics. The professional market area should be concerned with the "selling" of services that require a physician's recommendation, for example, surgery, cardiac rehabilitation, and anesthesiology. This area would also market the sale of hospital services, such as wellness programs to businesses, physical examinations for executives, and preferred provider organizations. The ultimate purpose of the persons in charge of these functions is to "configure the service so that it meets consumer needs better than the competitor's services and does so at a profit . . . Any marketing manager with product marketing responsibilities focuses first on the market, not the product" (Beckham, 1984). Such an industrial approach needs the full support of the CEO.

Market Research

Two of the marketing functions defined by Campbell (1981) — program research and evaluation functions and marketing information system functions — are generally grouped together under the umbrella designation of *market research*. However, it is necessary to distinguish between the two components of market research: *marketing information* and *market research*. "The distinction between general marketing information and market research is that the former can be collected and analyzed internally at little cost on a continuing basis. In contrast, market research should be performed when needed information about specific issues cannot be obtained from the general marketing information" (Clarke and Shyavitz, 1981). Marketing information can be obtained by all hospitals, whereas market research is usually performed by market research professionals, with the help of top hospital management.

Marketing Information

The basis of the marketing effort is information. Most industries use a marketing audit to gather information. A marketing audit is "essentially a data base to guide marketing decisions. Its fundamental purpose is to examine systematically how well the organization is doing in its market relations" (MacStravic, 1980). A marketing audit "involves examining the entire scope of the organization's activities" and is essentially "an information gathering process" (Berkowitz and Flexner, 1978).

In general, marketing audits contain information in three categories (MacStravic, 1980):

- Behavior, which covers the organization's behavior toward its markets, and vice versa
- Impact of that behavior, which covers the effect of the organization's behavior on its markets and vice versa
- Causal factors, which are the demographic and psychographic characteristics affecting the situation

Figure 6-3, next page, provides a suggested procedure for a market audit that focuses on these three types of information. Samples of two other marketing audit forms are shown in figures 6-4 and 6-5, at the end of this chapter.

A marketing audit has the following purposes (Shuchman, 1959):

- It appraises the total marketing operation.
- It centers on the evaluation of objectives and policies and the assumptions that underlie them.
- It aims for prognosis as well as diagnosis.

Figure 6-3. Suggestions for Market Audit

Step 1. Identify the specific set of market transactions you want to audit—e.g., inpatient utilization by service.

Step 2. Identify the specific behaviors you're interested in measuring for both current and past years:

                                                                                      Current   Past Years

A. Patients
  admissions
  length of stay
  average daily census (ADC)
  variability of census (standard deviation)
  ancillary service use
B. Physicians
  number of admissions
  length of stay
  vacation timing
  ancillary service use
  numbers of physicians on staff

Step 3. Describe how you behave with respect to this market:

A. Patients
  number of people wait-listed
  average length of wait for admission
  number of patients placed in "wrong" units
  proportion of time unit was understaffed/overstaffed
  percent of meals served hot, on time, etc.
B. Physicians
  admitting privilege rules
  priorities
  perquisites
  percent of admissions delayed
  percent of surgeries cancelled
  emergency room coverage required
  committee responsibilities

Step 4. Evaluate current behavior and current direction of change in terms of hospital performance/success measures:

    occupancy rate
    lost patient days because
      of lack of beds
    total revenue this service
    total expenses this service
    total estimated lost revenue due
      to lost patients, if any

    revenue contributions to other
      services
    expenditure contributions to other
      services
    payments as percent of charges
    receivables rate

Step 5. Identify patients' demographic and psychographic factors of interest that might explain behavior or be focused on to change it.

Demographic: age, sex, race, income, health insurance coverage, employment, size of family, residence, family physician, religious preference

Psychographic: knowledge of hospital's services, attitudes toward quality, cost, personal aspects of care received, understanding of condition, feelings about doctors, nurses, hospital

---

Reprinted, with permission, from *Marketing Objectives for Hospitals*, by Robin E. MacStravic, © by Aspen Systems Corporation, 1980.

- It searches for opportunities and means for exploiting them as well as for weaknesses and means for their elimination.
- It practices preventive as well as curative marketing practices.

Marketing information should include information on the hospital itself and on the hospital's general environment and competition. Clarke and Shyavitz (1981) provide a thorough breakdown of the kinds of information (internal and external) that is useful for marketing purposes (see table 6-3, next page). They point out that many hospitals already have a wealth of marketing information available or easily accessible to management. Marketing information is not expensive to collect, can be updated easily once the data base is established, and can be collected and analyzed by the hospital's own staff (Clarke and Shyavitz, 1981).

One individual should be assigned the responsibility of preparing the first draft of the audit report. This person should understand that not all of the collected data will be useful or should be reported. The report should emphasize identification and analysis of trends across departments, functions, and marketing targets. It should look at familiar data from a new or different perspective and capture the essence of that data in order to give new direction to marketing strategies.

The audit report should be in narrative form with a minimum number of tables. Both hard (quantitative) and soft (qualitative) data should be incorporated into the report, as should figures and quotes that support a point without being pedantic or folksy. The report might be divided into five major sections: hospital strengths, weaknesses, data needs, short-term marketing recommendations, and long-term marketing recommendations. Draft copies of the report should be circulated to the CEO, marketing department, marketing committee (if the marketing function is organized in this way), and department directors for review and comment.

From that point on, compromise is the name of the game. Undoubtedly specific issues or recommendations, particularly if they require substantial change, will hit sensitive nerves. However, it is important to remember that the overall goal of the marketing process is a more efficiently run institution. In the interests of achieving this goal, unnecessary organizational conflict resulting from personality differences should be avoided, even if it means compromise on what appears to be rational, objective findings.

Market Research

Market research is an "original, objective, systematic (and usually professionally performed)" investigation of specific issues or topics (Clarke and Shyavitz, 1981). It is performed when needed information about specific problems or issues cannot be obtained from general marketing information. Its value, therefore,

Table 6-3. General Marketing Information

Internal	External
Census—aggregate and by service	Characteristics of the hospital's service area
Admissions/discharges	
by service (medical, surgical, pediatric, etc.)	age distribution
by diagnosis within service	income distribution
by physician	level of education
by source of payment	by religion (if applicable)
by patient origin by community	by culture or ethnic background (if applicable)
by source of referral (medical staff, emergency room, outpatient department, etc.)	by medical service usage rates (inpatient, ambulatory, emergency room)
by patient age	market size and growth rate
by average length of stay	natality and mortality statistics
	membership in HMOs (number of members in each HMO)
Medical staff	Profile of MDs in hospital's market area
aggregate number and by department	age
by credentials	specialty
by specialty	practice setting
by age	office location
by practice plans	admission rates
by office location	affiliations
by use of ancillary services and operating room	patients' origins
by admissions by diagnosis	credentials
by other hospital affiliations and percentage use of each other hospital affiliation	
by total hospital revenue generated	

(continued)

Table 6-3 *(continued)*

Emergency department utilization
   gross utilization
   by shift
   by time of year, day of week
   by source of payment
   by patient origin by community
   by type of diagnosis
   time in waiting area until patient treated
   percentage of EMS ambulance runs to emergency department
   patient origin by incidence of emergency
   by source of referral (walk-in physician, fire, police, etc.)
   percentage of emergency department patients who are admitted as inpatients

Ambulatory medical services utilization
   gross utilization
   by service
   by diagnosis
   by patient source
   by patient origin in community
   by source of referral
   by patient age
   percentage of ambulatory patients who admitted as inpatients

Financial information
   revenues by department
   expenditures by department

Gross index of patient satisfaction with all services
   from patient cards
   from hospital ombudsmen

Competitors
   numbers of beds
   occupancy by service
   service configuration
   characteristics of population served
   service expansion or alteration plans including major capital projects
   medical staff makeup
   prices

Planning regulatory and hospital reimbursement trends

Medical (clinical) practice trends (i.e., decreasing tendency to hospitalize children, increasing use of home health care, etc.)

Reprinted, with permission, from "Marketing Information and Research: Valuable Tools for Managers," by Roberta N. Clarke and Linda Shyavitz, in *Health Care Management Review*, 6(1):74, Winter 1981.

Chapter 6/Marketing

lies largely in providing information that is complementary to rather than duplicative of marketing information.

Market research is appropriate for a hospital if the following questions can be answered in the affirmative (Clarke and Shyavitz, 1982):

- Are there specific unanswered questions that need to be answered in order to handle current marketing problems and opportunities?
- Are these unanswered questions answerable through original, objective, and systematic market research?

Market research generally is used to generate information on perceptions, preferences, potential demand, and usage (Clarke and Shyavitz 1981) The key to meaningful market research is the ability to focus on a single, specific issue.

The questions most commonly asked by market researchers deal with low occupancy rates and low utilization of services (Clarke and Shyavitz, 1982). Other issues frequently addressed are patient financial-mix problems, patient age-mix problems, and the impact of new competition. Questions may be specific to the organization's situation: they may focus on the whole organization or on specific services.

Generally, the kinds of questions market research is called on to answer are the what-if, how, and why questions rather than who, what, when, and where questions. The best research efforts usually are designed to answer a number of specific questions on one issue. However, a variety of issues may be addressed in one research effort as long as all of the issues are directed at the same markets, for example, medical staff or patients (Clarke and Shyavitz, 1982).

An example of market research in a rural hospital is provided by Memorial Hospital of Taylor County, Medford, Wisconsin. The hospital's board of trustees conducted a county resident opinion survey on health care facilities in Taylor County and vicinity to answer the following questions (Arnett, 1982):

- How can the hospital and the clinic improve the quality of care and referral services?
- How can the hospital and the clinic expand their existing services and facilities to more effectively meet the health care needs of their service area?
- How can the hospital and the clinic become the hub of an efficient health care network?

The survey results provided the following information, which was useful to the hospital corporation in developing and implementing its long-range plan:

- Demographic analysis of the population in the service area
- Information about health care insurance coverage and financing sources
- Profile of the hospital's medical staff

- Evaluation of the public's perception of the hospital
- Review of perceived satisfaction with specific service characteristics
- Evaluation of the migration of patients to other nearby facilities and the services sought by those who changed primary care facillties
- Information on the services the area's population desired the corporation to provide

The difference between the perceptions of the service area respondents and their apparent lack of knowledge regarding professional staff, services, and equipment became the focus of the service identification aspect of the marketing program. The objectives set were to reestablish and cultivate the identity of the hospital as a primary care center, inform the public of the availability of services, provide the information necessary for the area's citizens to make informed decisions on seeking services at the hospital, and increase the utilization of services at the hospital.

A hospital should consider performing its own market research only if it has staff members with the necessary expertise to do so. The skills required include familiarity and experience in the following areas (Clarke and Shyavitz, 1981): experimental versus nonexperimental research designs; sampling procedures; qualitative versus quantitative research; questionnaire construction; interview techniques and interviewer qualifications; various statistical techniques; and data analysis, processing, and interpretation.

In an attempt to minimize costs, some hospitals have tried to conduct their own research, and some of these have encountered problems. First, there are often difficulties in remaining unbiased and objective in the way questions are chosen and asked. Second, some health care organizations have found it difficult to perform a reasonable analysis of the vast amounts of data collected. Third, some nonprofessional market researchers find it hard to keep market research separate from promotion. In other words, the distinction between "what will be?" (a legitimate research question) and "what should be?" (a predetermined policy statement) becomes blurred.

Many hospitals employ one or more individuals with research skills in fields such as operations management or planning (Clarke and Shyavitz, 1982). Unfortunately, these individuals are often mistakenly used as market researchers also. Although basis research methodologies are somewhat universal, specific knowledge of market research techniques is essential if reliable information is to be obtained.

If no one on the hospital staff has the necessary skills, the CEO can look to consultants for assistance. However, the CEO must realize that, because health care marketing is a hot topic, some consultants have jumped on the marketing bandwagon and have falsely promoted themselves as having the necessary skills to undertake market research. Hospitals must be able to distinguish between real and proclaimed market research skills and experience. The skills and attrib-

Chapter 6/Marketing

utes to look for in selecting a market research consultant are the following (Clarke and Shyavitz, 1982):

- Knowledge and understanding of the purposes and applications of qualitative and quantitative market research
- Expertise in a variety of research methodologies
- Substantial experience in the use of qualitative research
- Substantial experience in designing market research projects, including data collection instrument design
- Substantial experience in managing the data collection (field study, telephone survey, one-on-one interviews) aspects of market research
- Substantial experience in managing the data processing and analysis aspects of market research; strong statistical skills
- If possible, health care market research; if not, substantial experience in utilizing market research skills in a variety of industries

If a hospital must choose between a consultant with market research background or one with health care background, it would be better served to choose the market research consultant. Hospitals can always provide the health care orientation, but they often cannot provide market research skills.

Another point to consider is the matter of cost. Market research, if done properly, is not cheap. Any hospital considering a market research project should be prepared to allocate sufficient funds for the effort.

The administrator should recognize that market research does have several limitations (Clarke and Shyavitz, 1982):

- Research will not supply all the answers to all the important marketing questions. Some markets are inaccessible, some subjects are too sensitive, and some issues are too complex.
- Research may produce inconclusive results or insignificant findings, making it difficult to support decision making.
- Market research findings, particularly if they incorporate information on attitudes or perceptions, are apt to be time limited simply because individuals change their minds.

Market research is a valuable tool for hospital managers. However, to be of value, the research effort should be used appropriately and with an understanding of its benefits and limitations.

References

Arnett, G. Diversification in a small, rural hospital. *Small or Rural Hospital Report.* 1982 July-Aug. 6(4):3-4.

Beckham, Daniel. Positioning marketing in the hospital's power structure. *Trustee.* 1984 Aug. 37(8):22-26,36.

Berkowitz, E. N., and Flexner, W. A. The marketing audit: a tool for health service organizations. *Health Care Management Review.* 1978 Fall. 3(4):51-57.

Campbell, B. Establishing a marketing organization for hospitals. *Journal of Health Care Marketing.* 1981 Spring. 1(2):26-32.

Clarke, Roberta N., and Shyavitz, Linda J. Marketing information and market research: valuable tools for managers. *Health Care Management Review.* 1981 Winter. 6(1): 73-77.

_____. Market research: when, why and how. *Health Care Management Review.* 1982 Winter. 7(1): 29-34.

Fine, Seymour H. The health product: a social marketing perspective. *Hospitals.* 1984 June 16. 58(12):66-68.

Goldsmith, J. C. The health care market: can hospitals survive? *Harvard Business Review.* 1980 Sept. 58(5):100-112.

MacStravic, Robin E. *Marketing by Objectives for Hospitals.* Germantown, MD: Aspen Systems Corporations, 1980.

_____. *Marketing Health Care.* Germantown, MD: Aspen Systems Corporation, 1977.

MacMillan, Norman H. *Marketing Your Hospital: A Strategy for Survival.* Chicago: American Hospital Association, 1981.

Robinson, L. M., and Whittington, F. Brown. Marketing as viewed by hospital administrators. In: Cooper, Philip D., ed. *Health Care Marketing: Issues and Trends.* Germantown, MD: Aspen Systems Corporation, 1979.

Sanchez, Peter M. Health care marketing at the crossroads. *Journal of Health Care Marketing.* 1984 Spring. 4(2):37-43.

Seymour, Donald W. What PPS means for hospital marketing. *Hospitals.* 1984 June 16. 58(12):70-72.

Shuchman, A. The marketing audit: its nature, purposes, and problems. In: *Analyzing and Improving Marketing Performance, Report No. 32.* New York City: American Management Association, 1959.

Tucker, S. L. Integrating planning and marketing activities in hospitals. *Health Care Planning & Marketing.* 1981 Apr. 1(1):1-7.

Chapter 6/Marketing

Figure 6-4. The Marketing Audit

THE MARKET AND MARKET SEGMENTS

- How large is the territory covered by your market? How have you determined this?
- How is your market grouped?
  — Is it scattered?
  — How many important segments are there?
  — How are these segments determined (demographics, service usage, attitudinally)?
- Is the market entirely urban, or is a fair proportion of it rural?
- What percentage of your market uses third party payment?
  — What are the attitudes and operations of third parties?
  — Are they equally profitable?
- What are the effects of the following factors on your market?
  — Age
  — Income
  — Occupation
  — Increasing population
  — ⟩ demographic shifting
  — Decreasing birthrate
- What proportion of potential customers are familiar with your organization, services, programs?
  — What is your image in the marketplace?
  — What are the important components of your image?

THE ORGANIZATION

- Short history of your organization:
  — When and how was it organized?
  — What has been the nature of its growth?
  — How fast and far have its markets expanded?
  — Where do your patients come from geographically?
  — What is the basic policy of the organization? Is it on "health care," "profit"?
  — What has been the financial history of the organization?
    — How has it been capitalized?
    — Have there been any account receivable problems?
    — What is inventory investment?
    — What has been the organization's success with the various services promoted?
- How does your organization compare with the industry?
  — Is the total volume (gross revenue, utilization) increasing, decreasing?
  — Have there been any fluctuations in revenue? If so, what were they due to?

(continued)

Figure 6-4 *(continued)*

- What are the objectives and goals of the organization? How can they be expressed beyond the provision of "good health care"?
- What are the organization's present strengths and weaknesses in:
  — Medical facilities
  — Management capabilities
  — Medical staff
  — Technical facilities
  — Reputation
  — Financial capabilities
  — Image
- What is the labor environment for your organization?
  — For medical staff (nurses, physicians, etc.)?
  — For support personnel?
- How dependent is your organization upon conditions of other industries (third-party payers)?
- Are weaknesses being compensated for and strengths being used? How?
- How are the following areas of your marketing function organized?
  — Structure
  — Manpower
  — Reporting relationships
  — Decision-making power
- What kinds of external controls affect your organization?
  — Local?
  — State?
  — Federal?
  — Self-regulatory?
- What are the trends in recent regulatory rulings?

COMPETITORS

- How many competitors are in your industry?
  — How do you define your competitors?
  — Has this number increased or decreased in the last four years?
- Is competition on a price or nonprice basis?
- What are the choices afforded patients?
  — In services?
  — In payment?
- What is your position in the market—size and strength—relative to competitors?

(continued)

Figure 6-4 *(continued)*

PRODUCTS AND SERVICES

- Complete a list of your organization's products and services, both present and proposed.
- What are the general outstanding characteristics of each product or service?
- What superiority or distinctiveness of products or services do you have, as compared with competing organizations?
- What is the total cost per service (in-use)? Is service over/under utilized?
- What services are most heavily used? Why?
  - What is the profile of patients/physicians who use the services?
  - Are there distinct groups of users?
- What are your organization's policies regarding:
  - Number and types of services to offer?
  - Assessing needs for service addition/deletion?
- History of products and services (complete for major products and services):
  - How many did the organization originally have?
  - How many have been added or dropped?
  - What important changes have taken place in services during the last ten years?
  - Has demand for the services increased or decreased?
  - What are the most common complaints against the service?
  - What services could be added to your organization that would make it more attractive to patients, medical staff, nonmedical personnel?
  - What are the strongest points of your services to patients, medical staff, nonmedical personnel?
  - Have you any other features that individualize your service or give you an advantage over competitors?

PRICE

- What is the pricing strategy of the organization?
  - Cost-plus
  - Return on investment
  - Stabilization
- How are prices for services determined?
  - How often are prices reviewed?
  - What factors contribute to price increase/decrease?
- What have been the price trends for the past five years?
- How are your pricing policies viewed by:
  - Patients
  - Physicians
  - Third-party payers
  - Competitors
  - Regulators

(continued)

Figure 6-4 *(continued)*

PROMOTION

- What is the purpose of the organization's present promotional activities (including advertising)?
  - Protective
  - Educational
  - Search out new markets
  - Develop all markets
  - Establish a new service
- Has this purpose undergone any change in recent years?
- To whom has advertising appeal been largely directed?
  - Donors
  - Patients
    - Former or current
    - Prospective
  - Physicians
    - On staff
    - Potential
- What media have been used?
- Are the media still effective in reaching the intended audience?
- What copy appeals have been notable in terms of response?
- What methods have been used for measuring advertising effectiveness?
- What is the role of public relations?
  - Is it a separate function/department?
  - What is the scope of responsibilities?

CHANNELS OF DISTRIBUTION

- What are the trends in distribution in the industry?
  - What services are being performed on an outpatient basis?
  - What services are being provided on an at-home basis?
  - Are satellite facilities being used?
- What factors are considered in location decisions?
- When did you last evaluate present location?
- What distributors do you deal with? (e.g., medical supply houses, etc.)
- How large an inventory must you carry?

Reprinted, with permission, from "The Marketing Audit: A Tool for Health Service Organizations, by Eric N. Berkowitz and William A. Flexner, in *Health Care Management Review*, 3(4):55-56, Fall 1978.

Chapter 6/Marketing

Figure 6-5. A Sample Marketing Assessment/Audit

What follows is a marketing assessment, or audit. This questionnaire is to be filled out by a CEO, or his/her designee. Its intent is to elicit some preliminary information and also to get some thinking started.

Respondents are asked to fill out the questionnaire as completely as possible, but not to worry if there are questions that cannot be responded to at the time.

1. **Marketing Decision-Making Apparatus**

    A. Who in the hospital do you think will set the hospital's marketing strategy and make the big decisions?

    The CEO? _____

    A board committee? _____

    A vice-president of marketing? _____

    Other? Please describe. _____

    _____

    B. Who in the hospital do you expect to be the main initiators of marketing actions?

    The CEO? _____

    A board committee? _____

    A vice-president of marketing? _____

    Someone else in the community? _____

    Who? _____

    The HSA? _____

    Other? Please describe. _____

    C. Who else do you expect to participate in the hospital's marketing decision-making process? Please describe.

    _____

2. **Use of Outside Consultants vs. Doing the Work In-House**

    Marketing is generally thought to encompass a number of specialist areas, listed below. Please indicate which of these activities you would expect to do in-house and those services you would expect to hire from outside the organization.

(continued)

Marketing/Chapter 6

Figure 6-5 (continued)

Marketing Specialty	In-House Activity	Service Hired Outside
Development of marketing strategy	_____	_____
Marketing management	_____	_____
Research of consumer attitudes about our hospital	_____	_____
Research of physician attitudes about our hospital	_____	_____
Public relations	_____	_____
Internal publications	_____	_____
Design and graphics	_____	_____
Advertising	_____	_____

3. **Priorities**

   Question 2 listed the activities that are generally thought to be part of marketing. Here is the same list. Please indicate the areas for which you feel the greatest sense of urgency. Do this by placing the number 1 after the activity of greatest urgency, 2 after the item of next greatest urgency, and so forth.

   Development of marketing strategy _____

   Marketing management _____

   Research of consumer attitudes about our hospital _____

   Research of physician attitudes about our hospital _____

   Public relations _____

   Internal publications _____

   Design and graphics _____

   Advertising _____

4. **Making Things Happen**

   Once the decisions are made, whom do you expect to be involved, on an ongoing basis, with implementing the decisions—making things happen? Some possibilities are listed below. Please indicate how you see them being employed.

   A. The hospital's public relations department _____

   B. The administrative staff _____

(continued)

Chapter 6/Marketing

Figure 6-5 *(continued)*

    C. A marketing manager hired from outside _____

    D. Volunteers _____

    E. An outside consumer research firm _____

    F. An outside public relations firm _____

    G. An outside advertising agency _____

    H. Others. What other thoughts do you have? _____

5. **Budget**

    What budget do you see being made available for marketing activities over the next five years?

    $$\$XXX$$

        Year 1 _____

        Year 2 _____

        Year 3 _____

        Year 4 _____

        Year 5 _____

6. **Sources of Information**

    A. Although marketing techniques have been used extensively by business for many years, they have not been widely used by hospitals. How did you first hear about marketing?

    B. How do you expect to keep abreast of the marketing field?

7. **Issues and Objectives**

    With what issues at your hospital do you expect marketing to be most helpful?

        Issue 1. _____

(continued)

Figure 6-5 *(continued)*

   Issue 2. _____
   _____
   _____

   Issue 3. _____
   _____
   _____

   What objectives will you set for the marketing activities of your hospital?

   1. _____
   2. _____
   3. _____

8. **Mission and Long-Range Plan**

   Marketing should serve the needs of the hospital's long-range plan. It should express the hospital's mission statement and make it "live." Please attach the hospital's

   - Mission statement
   - Long-range plan

9. **Data**

   A. Please describe or, if possible, attach any consumer research done for the hospital.
   _____
   _____

   B. Please describe or attach any data you have about physicians' attitudes toward the hospital.
   _____
   _____

   C. Please describe or attach any consumer research done to compare this hospital with alternative consumer choices, such as health maintenance organizations, surgery centers, and so on.
   _____
   _____

(continued)

Figure 6-5 *(continued)*

D. Please describe or attach any studies done by government agencies that might be pertinent to your marketing effort.

_____

_____

E. Please attach a map of the hospital showing its location and the location of competitive hospitals or alternative sources of treatment.

F. Please attach a list of each of your competitors showing
  - Total number of beds in use
  - Number of beds assigned to each department
  - Percentage utilization of each department for past five years

G. Please attach an assortment of the hospital's internal forms.

H. Please attach a complete package of any forms, letters, letterheads, brochures, or pamphlets that patients have seen in the past 12 months.

I. Please enclose snapshots or slides showing the hospital's interior and exterior signs.

J. Please enclose any advertising that your hospital has placed in the media (like newspapers) in the past three years. (If broadcast media were used, enclose the scripts.)

K. Please enclose "clips" of any articles about your hospital that have appeared in the past year.

10. **Other**

  A. In your opinion, what data should be asked for? Please list.

  _____

  _____

  B. What other questions should have been asked? Please write them down.

  _____

  _____

  C. Which questions need reworking to make them easier to understand and respond to?

  _____

  _____

Reprinted, with permission, from *Marketing Your Hospital: A Strategy for Survival*, by Norman H. McMillan, © by American Hospital Publishing, Inc., 1981.

Chapter 7
Diversification: Response to Community Need

Sandra L. Weiss
Donald F. Phillips

Hospitals must actively explore the many options available to protect and increase their market share and develop new sources of revenue. One strategy for accomplishing this end is diversification.

In financial terms, *diversification can be defined as* "the investment of the hospital's resources or the use of its economic clout to develop new sources of nonoperating revenues that are protected from regulation and reduction in reimbursement" (Gilbert, 1980). In broader terms, "diversification as practiced by the small and rural hospital is a conscious attempt on the part of this health care provider to expand the range of services provided in the community in order to meet the community's needs while at the same time optimizing the utilization of the full range of the hospital's organizational resources, thus providing a stable financial base and giving the hospital organization its greatest chance for survival" (Golda, 1981).

Hospitals should consider diversification because it can:

- Allow for institutional growth by protecting existing markets and adding new markets
- Strengthen the patient referral base
- Increase the revenue base
- Promote more effective competition
- Strengthen access to capital
- Develop more comprehensive health care services
- Expand the power base
- Create momentum to attract talent and resources
- Strengthen providers' ability to be reimbursed for services

Chapter 7/Diversification: Response to Community Need

Often, the motivation for exploring diversification options comes when a financial crisis seems imminent. For example, for hospitals experiencing a poor cash flow or problems with staffing, census, or accounts receivable, diversification seems tempting as a means of resolving problems. However, even though diversification offers a promise for economic recovery, it should not be viewed as a cure for poor fiscal management.

The Diversification Array

One way to think about diversification is to examine the entire range of services required in a community. An expression of individual need is heard, witnessed, or called to the attention of a referral agent or source. This person or organization uses any number of processes to match the individual in need with the appropriate services. Up to this point, hospital involvement may be nonexistent or minimal; however, the hospital should at least explore its possible relationship with the referral agents and its capability of offering or facilitating the linkage arrangements. Examples could be the operating of monitoring equipment, maintaining an ambulance service, or conducting patient or community health education programs.

Services can be divided into three primary categories, with the understanding that overlap usually exists. Welfare services refer to the provision of the personal necessities of life: food, housing, clothing, and protection or security. Social services include those areas that help make an individual a productive and happy person within the community; examples of such areas are education, employment, retirement, recreation, and family services. Health services, though closely related to social and welfare services, refer to ongoing medical, health, and nursing care. Health services are further divided according to type of care provided; the scope of care (primary, secondary, and tertiary); and the setting in which care is rendered (institutional, community, and in-home). To generate ideas for diversification, various combinations of the services across service areas as well as within each service area can be explored. However, specific community needs must always be kept in mind.

Another way of thinking about diversification is to define it in terms of target markets, the types of services to be provided, and the settings in which the services will be provided (Golda, 1981). Target markets could include the elderly, adolescents, healthy persons, the sick, employees of local businesses, other providers, health maintenance organizations, government agencies, and agricultural cooperatives. Services can be grouped into a number of categories: custodial, palliative, curative, restorative, rehabilitative, detection, prevention, promotion, protection, as well as other kinds of services only indirectly related to health, such as management of nonhospital facilities and parking lots. Service settings might include, besides hospitals, the home, long-term-care facilities, nursing homes, private physicians' offices, congregate care facilities, community

Diversification: Response to Community Need/Chapter 7

service centers, work place, freestanding clinics, mobile clinics, and community service clubs.

Diversification can take many forms. Hammer (1983) points out that "diversification can be 'related' through an expansion of the primary product line (health care) or 'unrelated' into areas not directly associated with the original line of business." Related areas could include the expansion of services within the hospital (hospices, swing beds, distinct-part long-term-care facilities, and family-centered care); ambulatory care facilities (primary care, satellite clinics, emergency and home care programs); health promotion activities (executive health and wellness programs); and other services such as mental health, family planning, rehabilitation services, and congregate housing. For each of these settings and programs, there are incentives and disincentives.

Related diversification can be vertical or horizontal (Wolford, 1981). "Under vertical diversification, the hospital may expand its product line by offering more comprehensive levels of health care through increased services." Some areas to be considered for vertical diversification are outpatient surgical unit, birthing centers, health maintenance organizations, partial hospitalization psychiatric centers, hospice care, skilled nursing facility, cardiac rehabilitation, commercial laboratory, emergency centers, ambulatory care centers, ambulance services, industrial medicine, executive fitness programs, and elderly housing. "Under horizontal diversification, the hospital diversifies, usually outside its immediate geographic service area, by expanding its operations to more than one hospital or health care entity." Some areas to be considered for horizontal diversification are hospital acquisitions (purchase or long-term leasing) and management contracts (for the entire hospital or a department).

Unrelated diversification can be as encompassing as the limits of imagination. Examples of unrelated types of diversification are ownership and construction of office buildings, medical or nonmedical; development of ambulance services; ownership of florist shops; selling of office equipment or laundry or catering and food preparation services; and the ownership of laboratories. "Unrelated diversification should not be pursued, however, without thorough review of the tax, reimbursement, and legal implications and the potential risks" (Hammer, 1983).

Diversification is one of the current buzzwords in the hospital industry. The concept of diversification seems to make sense, particularly in light of current economic conditions. However, hospitals, especially in rural settings, should approach diversification cautiously. For other industries, diversification usually means spreading their financial interests into other businesses. What hospital managers usually mean by diversification is the expansion of their product or service lines, not expansion into other businesses. The previously mentioned examples of non-health-care-related interests, such as real estate buildings, may work for major medical centers in urban areas that can afford the financial and personnel investments needed to spawn new businesses. Between four and seven

97

years are needed to solidly establish any new business, and there is no guarantee of returns on investments made.

The risks of diversification are evident even in the commercial world. Each year, hundreds of enterprises abandon unprofitable and unrelated businesses. The general lesson to heed is that few hospitals can afford to speculate on new services or businesses that are not directly related to their present ones. The soundest and safest way to grow is to find new uses for existing products and services, rather than to develop new products and services.

Organizational Responses to Options

Over the past several years, there has been sufficient experimentation in a variety of diversification efforts to acquire some insight into the problems associated with implementing new ventures. A guidebook on diversification alternatives for rural hospitals provides a step-by-step process to be used by hospital administrators and governing boards to meet the challenge of maintaining continued operation and also to explore innovative avenues to better the financial status, community service, and future outlook of their hospitals (Henning, 1980). The guidebook describes 37 alternatives, which are divided into three categories: *conversion,* in which beds are changed from one type of service to another or the number of beds is reduced in order to provide other services; *diversification with possible conversion,* in which the implementation of alternatives may or may not require space conversion; and *diversification,* in which no conversion is necessary. Table 7-1, at the end of this chapter, gives a brief overview of these 37 alternatives in terms of the following aspects: population served; need for renovation, delicensure, or certificate of need; reimbursement possibilities; advantages; and disadvantages.

Examples of some hospitals that have diversified in order to respond to declining census and consequently reduced revenues follow. These hospitals are also responding to the needs of their communities and have determined which types of diversification are most suited to the hospital and the community. Making such decisions requires careful analysis of the hospital's service area and the hospital's strengths and weaknesses.

Lake Chelan Community Hospital, a 28-bed, acute care, general hospital in rural north-central Washington, has diversified its services to include inpatient and outpatient psychiatric services, home health care, birthing room, and surgical services in an attempt to solve the hospital's historic low-occupancy problem (Peters and Tseng, 1983).

Northwoods Living Care Center, an 18-bed hospital in Phelps, Wisconsin, diversified into inpatient and nursing home care; children's day care; apartments for the elderly; youth programs; outpatient clinic; and three satellite clinics (Friedman, 1980, 1981; Kruse, 1985). One of these clinics is owned and staffed by the hospital, and the other two are affiliated with the hospital. The hospital is

Diversification: Response to Community Need/Chapter 7

located in a vacation area that also has a large retiree population. Its reasons for diversification were not only to gain a financial advantage but also to provide the community with needed services.

In January 1983, United District Hospital & Home in Staples, Minnesota, added home care service and in January 1984 began 14 additional services (Kuntz, 1984; Rice, 1985). United District has 40 acute care beds and a 100-bed nursing home. The new services added include adult day care and meals for senior citizens in the hospital's dining room on evenings, weekends, and holidays. The hospital has engaged an advertising agency to help it market its services. Although the hospital is in a competitive environment because of its closeness to Minneapolis and Duluth and because there are five other hospitals within 40 miles, its new ventures are beginning to be profitable.

Medford, Wisconsin, is a rural community of 4,500 persons and is the county seat of a farming and recreational area. Since 1962 when Memorial Hospital of Taylor County, Inc., was founded, the hospital has grown from 50 to 60 beds and continues to run the 104-bed nursing home it purchased in its first year of operation ("Diversification in a Small, Rural Hospital," 1982; Shulman, 1985; Arnett, 1985). The hospital has also purchased a medical office building, and it operates 10 efficiency apartments for residents who require some supervised care and a 24-unit retirement village for retirees who can live independently. In addition, the hospital provides substance abuse treatment and runs the county's ambulance service, an emergency medical technician training program, and a popular communitywide health education program that conducts wellness and physical fitness classes.

Smith County Memorial Hospital, Smith Center, Kansas, provides acute care services in its 26-bed facility and long-term care in its 28-bed facility to a service area of more than 5,000 persons in north-central Kansas (Erickson, 1985). Twenty-five percent of the population in this area is over 65 years of age. The hospital is operated under lease by Great Plains Health Alliance, Phillipsburg, Kansas, which is a multihospital system that contract manages or leases 26 hospitals (24 in Kansas, 1 in Nebraska, and 1 in Oklahoma). All of the hospitals in the system have fewer than 50 beds, and all but one are owned by governmental units. The system, which has been running hospitals since 1951, also provides hospitals with departmental services, such as accounting, strategic planning, marketing, physician recruitment, and data processing. Smith County Memorial Hospital, as well as other hospitals in the system, has diversified into many areas. The hospital has a swing bed program and distinct-part long-term beds. It operates the community's public health service, home health agency, school nursing program, and visiting hospice program.

Copley Hospital is the core of the Copley Health Systems, Inc., in Morrisville, Vermont (Friedman, 1983; Roberts, 1985). The hospital has 54 beds and is the sole provider in this rural northern Vermont area. Because the hospital is committed to serving the elderly, it set up a not-for-profit subsidiary that built

Chapter 7/Diversification: Response to Community Need

and operates Copley Terrace, a 38-unit housing development to provide elderly and handicapped persons with facilities for independent living. The housekeeping and maintenance services for these apartments are provided by hospital staff. Other subsidiaries include Stowe Health Center, Inc., an orthopedic facility that does business only on weekends during the ski season; Health Center Building, Inc., which owns and manages health offices; and Lifeline Foundation of Vermont, which provides home emergency medical alert systems to patients throughout Vermont and the other New England states. Stowe Health Center, Inc., and Health Center Building, Inc., are tax-paying corporations. In return for keeping rents low, the Health Center Building has restrictions in the leases that require the purchase of ancilliary services from the hospital. The hospital also markets and sells services to its subsidiaries and to corporations and hospital entities outside its system.

Sixty percent of Northwest Kansas Regional Medical Center's revenue comes from its many diversification activities. This 49-bed hospital is located in Goodland, Kansas, which is in the western part of the state, 17 miles from Colorado and 30 miles from Nebraska. The hospital operates a home health service and is developing policies for nonmedical supervised care, in which persons come to the hospital for flexible stays of from 1 to 14 days but are not formally admitted as inpatients. For example, elderly persons who are temporarily feeling unwell or unable to cope alone may stay overnight in the hospital, eat some meals at the hospital, and then return home; or they may stay in the hospital while their primary caretaker in the home is on vacation. The hospital is planning to build housing units for elderly persons who are able to live independently if they receive some help. Eighteen services, such as meals, maintenance, house cleaning, and lawn mowing, will be offered on a contract basis to persons living in these units. Since 1972, the hospital has operated a consulting program that consists of flying in specialists from Denver and Colorado Springs, Colorado, and from Hayes, Kansas. Fifty-five doctors participate in this program. The hospital has its own plane and pilot. Patients pay the hospital a flat fee that includes the use of the examination room and any support services and pay the doctors directly. Any surgery that is required as a result of these consultations is done at the hospital by the specialists. Among the other diversified services offered by the hospital are counseling and audiology, speech, physical, and occupational therapy; ambulance service for the county; migrant programs and programs for women, infants, and children for a seven-county area; meals for persons in their homes and meals for prisoners at the jail; Lifeline® program; and alcohol information and school for drunk drivers.

Many rural communities have a growing elderly population and a lack of available Medicare-certified nursing home beds. As a result, hospitals in these communities may look at swing-bed programs as a means of diversifying their revenue base and providing a needed community service. The term *swing bed* refers to a "hospital bed, usually in a small rural hospital, that can be used to provide acute care or long-term care" (Shaughnessy, 1984). The federal swing-bed eligibility requirements and the Medicare required standards for participation in the federal swing-bed program are discussed in *A Swing-Bed Planning Guide for Rural Hospitals* (Supplitt, 1984). The following hospitals are among 26 rural hospitals in Kansas, Mississippi, Missouri, New Mexico, and North Dakota who received grant money from the Robert Wood Johnson Foundation and its cosponsor, the American Hospital Association, to set up model swing-bed programs:

- Cedar County Memorial Hospital, a 34-bed hospital in El Dorado Springs, Missouri, is the sole health care provider in the community (Moomaw, 1985). A feasibility study confirmed the hospital's belief that a swing-bed program would benefit both the hospital and the community: the hospital could diversify its services and revenue base, and the community would receive needed long-term-care services. As a result of a decline in the hospital's occupancy rate, the hospital had the facilities and staff to provide the required skilled nursing care.

  An important task for Cedar County was educating the community and the hospital staff about the new service. As part of its marketing approach, the hospital set up a task force to promote a participative atmosphere among the medical staff, employees, and the community. The hospital developed a public relations program for clergy, community leaders, other health care providers, social service agencies, and others who might be working with patients who were to be part of the program. Informational pamphlets and a speakers' bureau were also part of the hospital's marketing efforts.

  When the program was implemented, Cedar County had to provide education and reinforcement for nurses and other personnel to help them accept their roles in the swing-bed program. Staff members had to understand that patients in adjacent beds would require different levels, or quantity, of care.

- The swing-bed program at Union Hospital in Mayville, North Dakota, has primarily private-pay patients who require skilled or intermediate nursing care (Salness, 1985). In North Dakota, the intent of swing-bed programs is not to keep patients more than 30 days. All the patients at Union Hospital are made aware of the hospital's commitment to short-term stays. Those patients who require care for a longer period know that they will be admitted to one of the two area nursing homes when space is available.

  Staff members at Union Hospital have been retrained to conduct the activities that hospitals participating in swing-bed programs must provide to increase the spiritual, psychological, and social well-being of their patients. As activites became established, the hospital received requests from discharged patients who wanted to come back to the hospital to participate in the activities program. These requests indicated that the community needed a geriatric day care center, and the hospital has instituted such a program.

Chapter 7/Diversification: *Response to Community Need*

For Union Hospital, the swing-bed program has resulted in a reduction of expenses and has provided a needed service to the community. The hospital was able to provide services without increasing the size of its staff.

Deciding to Diversify

Hospitals can look at the same circumstances and conditions that businesses use to determine whether they should diversify. Kotler (1976) points out that diversification is desirable for businesses under two general conditions: if a base business has increasing and excessive risk (competition, regulation, escalating costs) or offers less than desirable future growth and/or financial return and if the opportunities outside the base business are regarded as significantly superior. The for-profit business sector finds that diversification might be desirable under these circumstances (Kotler, 1976; Gluck, 1979; Salter and Weinhold, 1978; Leontiades, 1979):

- Current performance is marked by a slowdown in sales and earnings (for example, low utilization).
- Customer needs and demands are changing.
- The main product line has reached the mature phase of the business life-cycle.
- Excessive vulnerability to competition, regulation, and fluctuating demand exists.
- Swings of cyclical income streams are to be smoothed.
- A balanced portfolio where cash generators help finance cash takers is an established goal.
- Strengths and resources, such as management talent, physical facilities, and technology are underutilized.
- Capitalization on success in one locale through geographical expansion is desired.
- An entrepreneurial spirit and desire to grow exist.

In general, there are three areas to explore before any decision to diversify should be made: feasibility, regulation, and financing. The first area, making sure that the proposed change is feasible and well conceived, requires a rigorous strategic planning and marketing process. This is crucial for effective implementation of change. The marketing process should be a part of the overall institutional planning process and should be directly related to the hospital's mission. Within this planning and marketing process, the hospital must come to grips with its own strengths and weaknesses, determine what opportunities and threats it faces now and in the future, specify its own unique position and mission within the community, and define its goals and the strategies for achieving them.

Diversification: Response to Community Need/Chapter 7

The second area that needs attention before deciding on diversification options is the extent to which regulations, such as licensure, certificate-of-need, planning agency requirements, or other approvals, will affect the hospital's options. A thorough understanding of regulatory and payment programs is critical if new ventures are to succeed. As a general rule, it is easier to sell what the market wants than to get the market to buy what the organization wants to sell. To the extent that regulatory agencies view themselves as interpreters of the public need, they will generally take a more favorable position toward a hospital that proposes options in the public interest. Many of the regulatory programs, particularly those associated with the planning process, vary considerably from one part of the country to another and undergo much change over time. Therefore, hospitals at the local level should be aware of the prevailing attitudes and whims toward specific options and take advantage of the support that may emerge or be prepared for a lack of support. In addition, prior to taking any action that may have a legal or regulatory impact, hospitals should obtain appropriate advice from legal counsel.

The third area to examine before diversification decisions are made is the matter of financing. Before any decision is made, the following should have been done:

- A financial feasibility study should be under way or completed.
- The project should have the support of the governing board, administration, medical staff, and community.
- The payment schedule should be understood and should be adequate.
- The timing should be right.
- A market study should have shown a need for the program and community support for it.

Generally, hospitals have two sources of capital to fund new programs, facility improvements, and expanded services: internal operations, such as those obtained from depreciated funds and profits, and external equity and debt. As Hyde (1980) explains, the internal capital-generating capacity of hospitals has been deteriorating in recent years, because:

- The not-for-profit structure of most U.S. hospitals precludes generation of capital via investment.
- The tax laws of the United States have inhibited the receipt of philanthrophic gifts by hospitals.
- Increasingly stringent rate review policies restrict the hospitals' ability to seek competitive profit margins.
- Increasingly, cost-based reimbursement [as used in many state Medicaid programs] has failed to cover the full requirements of hospitals, and prospective pricing will not remedy this situation.

Chapter 7/Diversification: Response to Community Need

Financial Feasibility Study

Before any decision to diversify is made, a way must be found to sort out the institution's investment costs, risks, and expected returns. A basic question is what resource requirements, in terms of personnel, equipment, facility space and energy, finances, and patient load, are required to start up and maintain a new venture. The next question to ask is where the hospital can obtain these resources. The last question to ask is whether the hospital is going to develop its own resources or call on an existing organization to provide the resources.

Next, these resource requirements and project operations must be translated into dollars, with attention given to developing pro forma financial statements on capital and operating costs, including working capital, start-up costs, revenues and expenses, cash flow, estimates of amortization, and return on investment. Financial statements should be projected for at least three years of operation.

The hospital's outstanding debt and debt capacity should be determined as well as the impact of the venture on net cash flow and utilization of other hospital services. If capital is raised by refinancing, what effect will this have on the credit worthiness of the institution? The break-even point must be determined and analyzed in terms of financial needs and patient or service load.

Lewis (1981) suggests that hospitals apply sensitivity analysis to feasibility review by using a full range of scenarios, not just the most optimistic, in thinking through the impact of diversification. He urges hospitals to scale down optimistic projections by three degrees and apply Murphy's law: if anything can go wrong, it will.

Another aspect of sensitivity analysis is determining the risk that may occur by alienating competition in other areas. Friendly relationships with administrators of other institutions may suddenly cool off when the element of competition is introduced into the relationship.

Other problems to anticipate relate to what happens if diversification gets off to a slow start. How will a slow start affect cash flow? How will the hospital keep priming the pump? At what point will diversification be practically infeasible? On the opposite end of the scale, what happens if the hospital is more successful than anticipated?

Also, the hospital's opportunity costs, in terms of time and money, have to be considered when pursuing new interests. What other opportunities will be lost?

Another set of costs, one that Lewis (1981) believes is often forgotten, is what it costs to get out of a particular venture. What is the maximum downside risk, and how would the hospital go about salvaging capital expenses?

Last, quite aside from financial returns, are there other benefits, such as psychological boosts that encourage retention of talented staff or political gains, that place the hospital in a favorable position for other gains? These are some of the areas to consider when planning a feasibility review.

Because of the bleak outlook for capital financing of new ventures, the pressures for accountability to community needs, and the restrictions of regulatory bodies, a practical methodology for financial feasibility reviews that are agreeable to all parties needs to be developed. The basis for such a methodology may be the realization that the investment made by one hospital in a diversification effort influences the local health care economy and that decisions to support such efforts ultimately depend on the reassurance that the financial consequences would be favorable to the overall community, not just to the sponsoring hospital.

Evaluation

Once the decision to diversify has been made, the hospital must review its options. At this stage, criteria to evaluate various options must be developed. Each criterion should be weighted according to how valuable it is to the organization and how much compromise can be made with regard to an option meeting that particular criterion. The following are some criteria that might be used to evaluate diversification options (Hammer, 1983):

- Compatibility with existing business
  - Synergy
  - Degree to which there can be economies of scale
  - Common culture, values, management style
  - Potential negative impact on existing products and markets (for example, acceptance of medical staff, disruption to existing business)
- Size of the new activity
  - Relative to other services—should it be the dominant or supporting activity?
  - Resource requirement—capital intensive versus labor intensive
- Degree of freedom in the industry
  - Regulatory constraints—will a certificate of need be required?
  - Antitrust and other legal constraints
  - Pressure from special interest groups
  - Limitations of tax-exempt status
  - Licensure-accreditation requirements
  - Zoning requirements
- Market growth potential
  - Existing and potential competitors
  - Potential for geographic expansion
  - Increased market penetration
- Financial returns
  - Rate of return on investment
  - Amount of funds to be diverted from existing business
  - Cost of borrowing capital
  - Potential losses under worst-case situation

Chapter 7/Diversification: Response to Community Need

Once two or three options have been selected, a financial feasibility study can be conducted to determine the capital requirements, projected revenue and expenses, cash flow, and expected return on investment for each option. What constitutes an acceptable return on investment may vary from hospital to hospital. "Hospitals may elect to offer certain services to contribute to the community service base, improve the hospital's image, or increase referrals rather than solely for direct financial return" (Hammer, 1983). The hospital must carefully evaluate its reasons for wanting to become involved in each of the diversification options that they are considering.

Survival Strategy

Diversification is primarily a survival strategy, and rural hospitals can no longer afford to ignore either its potential or the pitfalls associated with it. Diversifying can help hospitals increase their revenue base and use their resources more efficiently and effectively. It can enhance the institution's image in the community, and this alone might be a good reason for a hospital to diversify as long as there is no increase in the operating costs of the hospital. After all, "maintenance and enhancement of public image are the cornerstone of any hospital's survival" (Golda, 1981). However, these activities can be detrimental to the hospital if they increase the operating costs of the hospital but do not produce revenue. "Diversification as a survival strategy applied to an institution that does not have its financial and administrative house in order may well hasten the day when the hospital must close" (Golda, 1981).

Hospitals considering diversification need to be aware that such actions require financial commitment and planning. It is important, therefore, "that the new business be compatible with the organization's basic management philosophy and style and match its culture" (Hammer, 1983).

In the development of this "new business," the importance of getting advice from legal counsel cannot be overemphasized, especially when the hospital is contemplating a departure from its traditional role as a provider of acute care. Diversification may require corporate reorganization. Among other things, hospitals will need to ensure that their tax status is maintained, that they are not violating antitrust limitations, that they meet the requirements of certificate-of-need regulations, and that they obtain the required licensure, accreditation, and zoning approvals.

Melum (1980) envisions three types of hospitals in the next decade: specialty centers, human services centers, and tertiary care acute hospitals. Specialty centers will focus on what they do best, such as pediatrics or crisis intervention. Tertiary care acute hospitals will provide more specialized tertiary care services than they do now and will be sites for research and continuing education. It is the human services centers that will be "most similar to the *reality* of hospital care in many rural communities. Human services centers of the future will be the focal point for broadly diversified human services. Some of these services will be typical acute services, but others will include such areas as fitness, counseling, employment services, personal care, nutrition, family planning, and other social services. This type of hospital organization will function as an *organizer* of human services for the community, as well as a provider of some of them. Many services will be offered on a prepayment basis." Diversification based on a market-oriented planning process can be the tool to help rural hospitals become the human services centers for their communities.

References

Arnett, Eugene W., president, Memorial Hospital of Taylor County, Medford, WI. Telephone conversation. 1985 June 20.

Diversification in a small, rural hospital. *Small or Rural Hospital Report.* 1982. 6(4):3-4.

Erickson, Curtis, president and chief executive officer, Great Plains Health Alliance, Phillipsburg, KS. Telephone conversation. 1985 July 16.

Friedman, Emily. Diversifying a rural hospital: a lot of work—and very rewarding. *Trustee.* 1981 Mar. 34(3):17-18, 20-21.

―――. Little hospital has big ideas. *Hospitals.* 1980 Nov. 16. 54(22):89-90.

―――. Sharing the wealth: rural hospitals can use corporate restructuring, Vermont administrator says. *Hospitals.* 1983 June 16. 57(12):88-91.

Gilbert, R. N. Organizational restructuring to accommodate diversification, growth and preservation of capital. Discussion paper, American Hospital Association Conference on Vertical Diversification through Development of Ambulatory Care, Chicago. 1980 Sept. 29.

Golda, E. A. Diversification: a survival strategy for rural hospitals. *Health Care Planning and Marketing.* 1981 July. 1(2):1-10.

Gluck, W. J. Planning growth through diversification. *Managerial Planning.* 1979 Jan. 27:1-6.

Hammer, L. Planning for hospital diversification. *Health Care Strategic Management.* 1983 Dec. 1(3):4-9.

Henning, C. *Alternatives for rural Hospitals.* Yankton, SD: Planning and Development District III, 1980.

Hyde, F. Capital consequences of diversifying: buildings, space and finance. Discussion paper, American Hospital Association Conference on Vertical Diversification through Development of Ambulatory Care, Chicago. 1980 Sept. 29.

Johns, L. Economic impact analysis: a theoretical approach. *American Journal of Health Planning.* 1977 Jan. 1(3):20.

Chapter 7/Diversification: Response to Community Need

Johns, L., Chapman, T., and Raphael, M. *Guide to Financial and Economic Analysis for Health Planning.* San Raphael, CA: Lester Gorsline Associates, 1975.

Jones, W. J. Selecting and implementing specific role options. In: Melum, M. M., editor. *The Changing Role of the Hospital: Options for the Future.* Chicago: American Hospital Association, 1980.

Kotler, Philip. *Marketing Management: Analysis, Planning and Control.* Englewood Cliffs, NJ: Prentice-Hall, Inc., 1976.

Kuntz, Esther F. Alternative services. Rural hospitals adding services to become healthcare centers. *Modern Healthcare.* 1984 Sept. 14(12):159-160, 162.

Kruse, Theodore F., administrator, Northwoods Living Care Center, Phelps, WI. Telephone conversation. 1985 June 20.

Laubach, P. B., and others. *Marketing Management for Health Care Executives.* Chicago: American College of Hospital Administrators, 1978.

Lewis, M. Speech presented at program on new options for small or rural hospitals. AHA Center for Small or Rural Hospitals. Portland, OR. 1981 Dec. 7.

Leontiades, Milton. Unrelated diversification: theory and practice. *Business Horizons.* 1979 Oct. 22:41-46

Melum, M. M., ed. Conclusion. *The Changing Role of the Hospital: Options for the Future.* Chicago: American Hospital Association, 1980, pp. 321-22.

Moomaw, Arlene. A swing-bed case study. *Small or Rural Hospital Report.* 1985 May-June. 9(3):unpaged insert.

Peters, J. P., and Tseng, S. *Managing Strategic Change in Hospitals: Ten Success Stories.* Chicago: American Hospital Publishing, Inc., 1983, pp. 155-57.

Rice, Tim, administrator, United District Hospital and Home, Staples, MN. Telephone conversation. 1985 June 19.

Roberts, Carolyn C. Diversification options for small and rural hospitals: a case study. Speech at session on diversification at the Eighth Annual Conference for Small or Rural Hospitals, conducted by the Section for Small or Rural Hospitals of the American Hospital Association, Chicago. 1985 June 6.

Salter, Malcolm S., and Weinhold, Wolf A. Diversification via acquisition: creating value. *Harvard Business review.* 1978 July-Aug. 56:166-76.

Salness, John. Presentation at session on swing beds at Eighth Annual Conference for Small or Rural Hospitals, conducted by the Section for Small or Rural Hospitals of the American Hospital Association, Chicago. 1985 June 6.

Shulman, Jan. Rural hospitals face upheaval. *Media Background Sheet,* prepared by the Department of Media Relations of the American Hospital Association, Chicago. 10 June 1985.

Shaughnessy, P. W. Overview of swing-bed care. In: Supplitt, J. T., ed. *A Swing-Bed Planning Guide for Rural Hospitals.* Chicago: American Hospital Publishing, Inc., 1984.

Shaughnessy, P. W., and others. *An Evaluation of Swing-Bed Experiments to Provide Long-Term Care in Rural Hospitals.* Vol. 1, *Final Summary Report.* Vol. 2, *Final Technical Report.* Denver: Center for Health Services Research, University of Colorado, 1980.

Supplitt, J. T. Swing beds: new diversification opportunity for small and rural hospitals. *Hospitals.* 1982 Nov. 16

_____, editor. *A Swing-Bed Planning Guide for Rural Hospitals.* Chicago: American Hospital Association, 1984.

Wilson, Bill D., administrator, Northwest Kansas Regional Medical Center, Goodland, KS. Telephone conversation. 1985 August 16.

Table 7-1. Diversification Alternatives for Rural Hospitals

Alternative	Population Served	Renovation Needed	Delicensure Needed	Con Needed	Reimbursement	Advantages	Disadvantages
CONVERSION							
1. Nursing Homes	Most elderly, some under 65 (10% of all nursing home residents are under 65. These include victims of multiple sclerosis, stroke, arteriosclerosis, broken bones, and other debilitating diseases and conditions)	Yes, to meet licensure standards	Yes	Yes	Medicaid, Medicare, state, county, private insurance, private pay	The same staff and service units will be used. Increased emphasis on long-term care with provisions of social and recreational activities will fill unmet need and provide continuum of care with shared services and cost-effectiveness.	Costs of renovation or construction may add capital expenditures that will reduce financial feasibility of switching to a lower level of revenue generation.
2. Psychiatric beds	Those persons in need of inpatient services based on psychological factors	No, unless to ensure security	No	Yes	Medicaid, Medicare, state, county, private insurance, private pay	Specifically trained staff can provide more comprehensive services than the existing approach of general medicine.	If a psychiatrist is not available, these services cannot be offered. Utilization may be low because stigma exists regarding specific designation of beds as psychiatric.
3. Detoxification	Those persons in need of detoxification services	No, unless to ensure security	No	Yes	Private pay, county, BC/BS group policy, private insurance, Division of Alcoholism contracts	Provide medical detox in the home community or close by. Provides place for care and treatment of the intoxicated person rather than incarceration and could provide first step to recovery.	Need specifically trained staff; stigma exists concerning hospitalization for intoxification; some difficulty may exist in reimbursement.

(continued)

Table 7-1 (continued)

Alternative	Population Served	Renovation Needed	Delicensure Needed	Con Needed	Reimbursement	Advantages	Disadvantages
4. Hospice	The terminally ill usually suffering cancer	Yes	Yes	Yes	Medicaid, Medicare, private pay, private insurance	Many people suffer from cancer; the rural agricultural areas have an incidence that is three times greater than urban. Hospice care will benefit these areas.	Utilization may be low because many people resist idea of going someplace to die. Thorough investigation needs to be conducted concerning attitudes toward hospice care and prevalence of terminal cancer in the area.
5. Adult day care	Those persons over 18 who for physical or mental reasons are unable to be left unattended	Yes	Yes	Yes	At present, varies from state to state, possible Title XX. In recent demonstration program, Part B Medicare was used to cover expenses.	Uses existing space to provide service that eliminates or lessens need for institutionalization.	May not be enough need for service in rural community. Careful assessment must be conducted. Reimbursement problems may limit the feasibility of the program.
6. Infant day care	Working parents with children under six months	Minimal	Yes	Depends on state law regarding closure of beds	Title XX and private pay	Use of existing staff to provide day care for infants will generate revenue and provide much-needed service for working parents.	Cost-of-care provision may not be regained through reimbursement, especially from Title XX which in South Dakota pays 55¢ per hour.

(continued)

Diversification: Response to Community Need/Chapter 7

Chapter 7/Diversification: Response to Community Need

Table 7-1 (continued)

Alternative	Population Served	Renovation Needed	Delicensure Needed	Con Needed	Reimbursement	Advantages	Disadvantages
7. Physician office	Service-area population	Yes	Yes	Depends on state law regarding closure of beds	Payment from physician for leasing of space and equipment	The attraction to new physicians is greatly enhanced by providing clinic and equipment on a lease basis. Additional physicians stimulate hospital utilization.	In rural areas physicians come and go, making it possible that the hospital may have periods where no rent is collected to make payments.
8. Dental offices	Service-area population	Yes	Yes	Depends on state law regarding closure of beds	Payment from dentist for leasing of space and equipment	The co-location of the dentist and hospital provides for dental services to the handicapped or those needing anesthesia.	The expense of setting up the practice may not be regained by leasing space and equipment. Careful assessment is mandatory.
9. Social services offices	Service-area population	Yes	Yes	Depends on state laws regarding closure of beds	Payment from social services for lease of space	The housing of social services within the hospital may facilitate the referral system between medical and social services.	The amount of payment may not warrant cost of renovation and overhead especially if services are part-time.
10. Nonhealth offices	Persons in need of office space; others dependent on use of office space	Yes	Yes	Depends on state law regarding closure of beds	Payment from lease	Steady income from unutilized space helps to cover overhead expenses.	Cost of renovation of rooms may exceed lease payments. Change to nonhealth status may change reimbursable costs. Thorough investigation of ramifications must be made.

(continued)

Table 7-1 (continued)

Alternative	Population Served	Renovation Needed	Delicensure Needed	Con Needed	Reimbursement	Advantages	Disadvantages
11. Medical clinic sponsorship on site	Service-area population	Yes, dependent on need of facility	Yes	Yes	Medicaid, Medicare, private insurance, private pay; federal grants also available to operate these.	Increases the capacity of the hospital to provide health services, generates revenue, and often increases the vitality of the hospital.	Increased administrative responsibilities, cost of renovation, staff, and equipment may not be recovered through revenues.
12. Dental clinic sponsorship	Service-area population and handicapped persons from the area.	Yes	Yes	Yes	Private insurance, private pay, Medicaid, developmental disabilities payments	Provides service to community and area, generates revenue, and meets special needs of handicapped.	Success depends on utilization, amount of revenue generated and the retention of dentist. Cost of renovation, equipment, and staff must be regained as it cannot be allocated elsewhere.
DIVERSIFICATION WITH POSSIBLE CONVERSION							
13. Satellite clinic sponsorship	Surrounding-area residents	Yes, if needed	No	Yes	Private insurance, private pay	Broaden service base; more accessible care means better health care and increased utilization of the sponsoring hospital.	More administrative duties; staffing may fluctuate and be too expensive to offer these services.
14. Children's handicapped medical needs	Mentally handicapped youth	Minimal, if any	Depends on space needs	Yes	School districts have a mill levy for special education, which is matched by the state to pay for these services.	Cost sharing would enhance the ability of the area to employ well-trained professionals, thereby bettering the health system.	School districts may not wish to part with control of these services (speech therapy, physical therapy, audiology). The level of services varies from one school district to another.

(continued)

Chapter 7/Diversification: Response to Community Need

Table 7-1 (continued)

Alternative	Population Served	Renovation Needed	Delicensure Needed	Con Needed	Reimbursement	Advantages	Disadvantages
15. Birthing rooms	Parents and newborns	Yes, but minimal	Possible	No	Medicaid, Medicare, private insurance, private pay	Enhance birth process, keep deliveries in the community.	Cost of renovation, furniture, and birthing bed when weighed against number of births may not be cost-effective.
16. Physical rehabilitation	Victims of cerebral palsy, muscular dystrophy, accidents, stroke, heart attack, arthritis, and rheumatism	Minimal; some equipment purchase	Depends on space requirements	Yes	Medicaid, Medicare, private insurance, private pay	Physical therapy is an important service for both inpatient and outpatient needs. Provision by the community retains some persons who would be transferred to other facilities.	The need for physical therapist must be evaluated prior to employing one because the salary may exceed the revenue generated.
17. Cardiac rehabilitation	Those persons who have suffered a myocardial infarction or bypass surgery or have coronary heart disease	Depends on size of program; some equipment purchase needed.	Depends on space needs	Yes	Medicare, some BC/BS plans, private pay	This program is easy to implement. Provides a real service to community residents by allowing people to participate in the home community.	A certain size of patient load is required to support this program. The size depends on costs.

(continued)

114

Diversification: Response to Community Need/Chapter 7

Table 7-1 *(continued)*

Alternative	Population Served	Renovation Needed	Delicensure Needed	Con Needed	Reimbursement	Advantages	Disadvantages
18. Alcohol and substance abuse counseling program	Persons in need of alcohol or drug counseling, spans all age groups and socioeconomic levels	Minimal	Depends on space requirements	Yes, if the hospital operates the program.	Title XX, NIAAA, NIDA, private pay, or lease payments	Many admissions to hospital are key to identifying chemical dependency, also the health status of the population is greatly affected by alcohol and substance abuse; thus a program such as this would be definite community service.	The amount of payment may not be commensurate with the cost of the program. However, if the hospital merely leases space for an outside agency to provide services on-site, this problem will be alleviated, and positive benefits can still be retained.
19. Mental health services	Those persons of all ages who are in need of outpatient counseling. This service is more widely used than ever.	Minimal	Depends on space requirement	Yes, if hospital operates the program	Title XX, NIMH, private insurance, private pay	A significant number of physical complaints have psychological causes. The interdependency of mental and physical health is clearly evidenced. The provision of mental health services in the hospital lessens visibility and heightens accessibility to the community.	A full-time counselor may be too expensive for the size of the program. A shared-service concept with other hospitals or leasing space to an existing agency will alleviate this problem.

(continued)

115

Chapter 7/Diversification: Response to Community Need

Table 7-1 (continued)

Alternative	Population Served	Renovation Needed	Delicensure Needed	Con Needed	Reimbursement	Advantages	Disadvantages
20. Congregate housing with support services	Those elderly or handicapped who are in need of some support services. Typical resident is white, middle class, female, and single widowed; 75% are 75 years or older.	Yes, or construction	Possible if existing space is renovated	Possible; depends on state regulations	Housing; FHA insured loans Section 231; Section 202 of Housing Act of 1959; Section 8 of Housing and Community Development Act of 1974, etc. Support Services: Administration on Aging, private pay, social services.	Shared-services concept works to allow flexibility in the amount of services provided while keeping costs to a minimum and retaining maximum amount of independency for resident.	There may not be enough need for this housing to warrant construction or renovation; administration will fall to hospital administrator; deals with a number of federal and state programs may be required, increasing paperwork and red tape.
21. Exercise and recreation programs	Can be available to everyone, especially successful in cases where special health problems exist	Possible	Possible	Possible	Private pay at present	Improve health status and health maintenance of population.	Cost of program may not warrant implementation.
22. Health promotion and wellness	Entire population	No	No	Possible	Private pay, contracts with employers	Hospital's role includes more than care of the sick. Healthy state of community benefits hospital.	No third-party payers may hinder success of program unless local business can offer it as a fringe benefit to employees or there is significant community commitment.

(continued)

Table 7-1 (continued)

Alternative	Population Served	Renovation Needed	Delicensure Needed	Con Needed	Reimbursement	Advantages	Disadvantages
DIVERSIFICATION							
23. Swing beds	Mostly elderly, some persons under 65 (10% of all nursing home residents are under 65; these include victims of multiple sclerosis, stroke, arteriosclerosis, broken bones, and other debilitating diseases and conditions)	No	No	Yes	Medicare, Medicaid, state, county, private insurance, private pay	Ability to switch usage, utilize same staff, generate revenue.	Unless attached to a nursing home, many social and recreational services may be lacking.
24. Seasonal outreach clinics	Tourists, migrants, isolated residents	Possible, depends on whether a mobile unit is used or an existing building	No	Yes, if operated by hospital and no outpatient services offered in past 12 months	Medicare, Medicaid, county, private insurance, private pay	Provide services to those in need, generate revenue, increased utilization of hospital as indicated, provide accessible emergency care.	Cost of services may be too high to warrant provision. Mobile unit is costly and may not pay for itself if used on seasonal basis. Renovation costs may have same drawbacks.
25. Indian health service	Indian tribes in area	No	No	No	100% cost reimbursement for IHS; contract or fee for service with Tribe under Self-Determination Act	Contract guarantees payment, Indian need for health services is greater than average, provides necessary services for Indian population in absence of IHS hospital.	Success depends on relationship with tribe, proximity to reservation, and past experiences of hospital contracts with the tribe.

(continued)

Table 7-1 (continued)

Alternative	Population Served	Renovation Needed	Delicensure Needed	Con Needed	Reimbursement	Advantages	Disadvantages
26. Industrial health service contracts	Employees of local industries and their families	No	No	No	Contracts with industries	Direct contracting cuts out middleman and ensures hospital of steady income.	Cost of services may exceed amount of contract or not be competitive with regular insurance programs.
27. Home health care	Sick or disabled homebound persons	No	No	Yes	Medicare, Medicaid, Title XX, some private insurance, private pay	Home health care provision is excellent follow-up to inpatient care.	Home health care reimbursement may vary from state to state. In some states, home health care is a statewide program operated by state government precluding the development of private agencies.
28. Public health services	Service-area population	No	No	Questionable	State, county, Medicare	Community service and integration of health services.	Political climate is extremely important in this case. Counties may be very protective of control.

(continued)

Table 7-1 (continued)

Alternative	Population Served	Renovation Needed	Delicensure Needed	Con Needed	Reimbursement	Advantages	Disadvantages
29. School health nursing	School-age children 5-18 years old	Minimal if any	No	Questionable	Contracts with school districts	Utilize existing staff or employ nurse part-time in both hospital and school. Cost sharing should allow more efficiency of operation.	The school nurse and school health program may amount to more work than money, especially since the cost of administration is shifted from school to hospital and may not be paid for. The specifics of the school health program vary from district to district and from state to state. Careful study must be made to ensure beneficial aspect of providing this service.
30. Community health education	Entire population	No	No	No	Health-risk education grants from the Center for Disease Control in Atlanta, GA; Possible monies from Department of Education in form of community education grants; community and county may provide funds	Improve health status and health maintenance of area residents.	Competitive nature of funding may preclude implementation of this project.

(continued)

Chapter 7/Diversification: Response to Community Need

Table 7-1 (continued)

Alternative	Population Served	Renovation Needed	Delicensure Needed	Con Needed	Reimbursement	Advantages	Disadvantages
31. Circuit-riding specialists	Entire population	No	No	No	Title XVIII, Title XIX, private insurance, private pay	Group practice of specialists providing circuit riding services to one or more rural hospitals would help keep down number of transfers, keep occupancy level up, and better the health care services in the area. Also, provide professional exchange and consultation thus, creating happier environment for family practice physician located in community.	Sufficient utilization must exist in order to support cost of specialists, which may be handled either as fee-for-service or on a contractual basis.
32. Cross-trained personnel	Service-area population	No	No	No	Significant savings will arise from employing one person who performs two or more roles in the hospital.	Having persons on hand cross-trained in areas such as pharmacy, anesthesia, respiratory therapy, speech therapy, X-ray, lab, EKG, administration, etc. provides a cost-effective means of providing services.	Careful consideration should be given to not overloading an employee who might quit and leave two or more vacancies. Paying for further training is feasible only when the cost-benefit ratio justifies this expense.

(continued)

Table 7-1 *(continued)*

Alternative	Population Served	Renovation Needed	Delicensure Needed	Con Needed	Reimbursement	Advantages	Disadvantages
33. After-hours communication center	Service-area population	No, but equipment may need to be purchased	No	No	Contracts with county and city governments	Complete utilization of staff. One basic place to call for everything: fire, ambulance, emergencies, law enforcement, etc.	Staff requires training. Some equipment may need to be purchased.
34. Expanded pharmacy services; mail-out prescriptions; delivery service	Isolated residents	No	No	No	Customary reimbursement for prescriptions with slight delivery charge	If a pharmacy department already exists, the expansion of this service could prove beneficial to isolated rural residents or those that are homebound.	This service may not work if it is in competition with other pharmacies because a significant amount of business loss might force druggist to leave town, lessening the services available to community residents.
35. Expanded laboratory	Service-area population	Possible; equipment may need to be purchased	No	No	Medicaid, Medicare, private insurance, private pay	If a substantial amount of lab work is "farmed out," it could be financially beneficial to invest in equipment to perform more lab work for the area physicians.	The utilization level of the new equipment and the cost of further training may not be covered by the increased revenue. Careful study of records must be done to ensure reasonable projections.

(continued)

Chapter 7/Diversification: Response to Community Need

Table 7-1 (continued)

Alternative	Population Served	Renovation Needed	Delicensure Needed	Con Needed	Reimbursement	Advantages	Disadvantages
36. Dietary services; Meals on Wheels; special diet preparation; dietetic consultation; meals for county jail; large-meal preparation (catering service)	Area residents	No	No	No	Varying sources depending on type of service: Office on Aging, county funds, private pay	Because the kitchen is already in use and cost of preparation becomes minimal in larger quantity, these services should generate a fair amount of additional income.	Cost of providing services may exceed reimbursement if the different programs overload the administrator and require hiring additional staff.
37. Laundry services; commercial laundry for motels and restaurants; diaper service	Area population, businesses requiring laundry services, families with children in diapers	No	No	No	Private pay	Because laundry may be underutilized, expanded use is feasible and may be profitable. Diaper service would ensure the complete sterilization and sanitariness necessary for diapers at a cost lower than disposable diapers.	In case of diaper service, the demand must be present because delivery service is almost a must. The commercial laundering may not pay for itself and provide headaches for administrators.

Reprinted, with permission, from *Alternatives for Rural Hospitals*, © Planning and Development District III, Yankton, SD, 1980, pp. 19-27.

Chapter 8

Management Options

Montague Brown
Barbara P. McCool

Introduction

In many states, headlines proclaim "University Medical Center Sells Out to Hospital Chain," with the accompanying article stating, "With the sale of this major medical center, investor-owned hospitals and their national insurance organizations have become leading health care providers in the state." Sound farfetched? Such changes in ownership, commonplace with smaller hospitals, now open the possibility that major companies will become providers in all sectors of the health care economy.

Consider the following. A 30-bed rural hospital built with Hill-Burton funds sells out to a chain organization headquartered in a major city 1,000 miles away. A 500-bed county hospital contracts with a management company to provide advice and consultation. A county commission signs a $3.5 million yearly lease for its 450-bed hospital, which last year earned more than $4 million after expenses. A 60-bed voluntary hospital hires a management company (owned by a religious order) to run it. A local voluntary hospital announces that it has contracted to manage a hospital in another town. Another hospital announces that it is acquiring an institution in another state. What do all these events have in common? Is any single hospital immune to these changes?

Whether a community wishes to afford itself the opportunities represented by multihospital systems is a choice, not an inevitability. At the same time, it is a choice that must be made explicitly. These new firms will inevitably approach every attractive business opportunity in the country, and so the governing board and management of every hospital must carefully consider how they should react.

Adapted and updated from *Management and Ownership Options for Independent Hospitals: A Decision Maker's Guide,* by Montague Brown and Barbara P. McCool. © 1983 by the American Hospital Association.

123

Chapter 8/Management Options

During the past decade, the organization and ownership patterns of hospitals changed dramatically. National hospital management companies grew from relative obscurity to multibillion-dollar enterprises with growth rates of 20 to 30 percent per year. Not-for-profit church and community-owned hospital organizations also began to develop chain-type operations or rushed to develop regional systems consisting of hospitals and other health care services. In addition, some of the more traditional shared services organizations, which are owned or operated in a manner similar to farm cooperatives, developed the capability to provide management services for local owners. In recent years, these shared services organizations have also begun leasing and owning hospitals.

As a result of these changes, hospitals became hot property, eagerly sought by aggressive salespeople. Although such readily available help may be a welcome change from the past, hospitals should proceed cautiously when deciding issues central to a vital community service. Because a lease and, sometimes, a contract to manage can be nearly as permanent and complete a separation of community control as a sale, a thorough review of the options by those with fiduciary responsibilities seems necessary and prudent.

However, with the strong downturn in hospital occupancy beginning in 1984, some hospitals have already become unattractive to any buyers. Until this time, the issue for potential sellers was whether or not to sell and to whom. Buyers were plentiful. Now potential buyers are beginning to question more closely whether buying at any price is feasible. With the industry facing occupancy rates of 50 percent or less, some hospitals are simply not going to be needed.

In spite of this environment, there are numerous new competitors interested in providing services and managing hospitals. This situation may be good for hospitals because these aggressive new organizations—regional hospital systems, national chains, and investor-owned, religious-sponsored, and other not-for-profit organizations—provide some opportunities to community hospitals to lease, sell, or contract for full management.

This chapter assumes a middle course between doing nothing and selling the hospital. New opportunities may represent progress or not, depending on how carefully each community deals with the organization that is bidding to become its local hospital owner or manager. If the community chooses to turn the operation over to an outside firm, that is a community decision. However, community leaders can benefit from a thorough review of the issues and likely implications of each form of organizational change.

What, for example, are some of the major problems that lead trustees, county commissioners, traditional religious sponsors, and others to consider selling, leasing, or hiring a management firm to take on the role normally played by an individual hospital administrator? What do these new firms, and older ones offering new services, represent? How do they differ, and what do they seek in a relationship? What is the nature of the various business agreements possible? How do they differ from some of the more traditional approaches to helping

Management Options/Chapter 8

the single hospital gain outside expertise, capital, and other resources? What questions should prudent trustees, public officials, or others responsible for the institution's best interests ask when considering contract management, lease, or sale of the hospital to another firm? Are there any potentially unanticipated consequences that should be considered in these deliberations? These and other such questions are the subject of this chapter.

Although much of this chapter discusses issues related to having outside organizations perform significant management and ownership roles in community hospitals, it is neither essential nor inevitable that these hospitals lose total control over their destiny. Many small hospitals can remain vibrant community institutions with good trusteeship, sound management, and liberal use of resources from a variety of sources, including government, universities, hospital associations, and consulting, accounting, and law firms. Shared services organizations can provide these hospitals with a variety of needed services not readily available to single institutions. Also, new organizations, ranging from simple shared laundries to wide-ranging organizations similar to the large farm cooperatives that serve small and large farmers, are continuing to develop their services.

Pressures on Rural Hospitals

With the advent of prospective pricing, intensifying competition, and new consumer and insurance demands for information on provider costs, rural hospitals will never again be the same. They must adapt and transform themselves to survive.

Today many medical and surgical procedures can be safely offered at lower cost in ambulatory settings. Although these new services are applauded by policymakers, they mean that hospitals will now face new and stiff competition from their own or former medical staffs. Such issues will undoubtedly influence trustees as they look at their hospitals' long-term future and question which approach they should take to ensure the security of their community's health care resources. Hospital strategies should not be isolated from physician strategies for the total community.

Technological advances and improved equipment, methods, and devices continue to put heavy pressure on hospitals to keep up to date. Administrators know that they must keep pace not only to serve patients but also to continue to attract physicians, who naturally prefer to admit patients to a full-service, modern institution. Cost containment pressures alone make this situation increasingly difficult. Keeping up and continually modernizing also places heavy strains on the capital potential of hospitals and makes them vulnerable to buy or lease offers. Government-owned hospitals are especially ripe for such offers, because the alternatives to selling or leasing may be a tax increase or governmentally guaranteed bond financing at high interest rates.

Chapter 8/Management Options

Hospitals will have great difficulty in getting the necessary capital to replace aging plants (often built with Hill-Burton funds) and to move into new program areas, such as long-term care, housing for the elderly, and emergicenters. Difficulty does not mean impossibility, nor does it mean that needed institutions will close. It does, however, call for a serious assessment of an institution's capital formation needs over a long-term period. Explicit steps should also be taken to ensure that, as capital problems arise, specific actions will be undertaken to meet the needs of the community.

There are several reasons why observers predict a capital crunch for hospitals. The capital markets, especially the tax-exempt markets, are highly competitive, making access to them much more difficult and impossible for weak institutions. Yet, even under the best of circumstances, many small, single, private and publicly owned hospitals get relatively poor ratings for borrowing. In addition, many hospitals manage to earn little or nothing; depreciation is not funded but spent for operations, thereby leaving such institutions without easy access to capital.

Hospitals can be managed in a manner that keeps them responsive to public needs and sufficiently profitable so that they will be better candidates for the capital they need to remain viable community hospitals. The fact that companies offer to manage, lease, or buy such operations indicates that these hospitals can be successful. Even some hospitals that should not continue to exist are finding themselves the objects of sales efforts.

Public tax revolts and the political aftermath of such problems add another dimension to health care trends. Although all hospitals are susceptible to these pressures, public hospitals are especially vulnerable. Local officials sense that cutbacks in federal and state support for medical care will ultimately affect the fiscal integrity of their hospitals. Because these same cities and counties already spend heavily for health care, any new burdens are especially troublesome.

Moreover, rural and small hospitals that were built with Hill-Burton funds may now need to replace or renovate their facilities. Some of these hospitals are still "repaying" their federal grants by providing mandated uncompensated care. Operational dollar cuts also loom large, and there are no federal bailout funds to replace aging facilities. Because many public hospitals have such policies as spending depreciation dollars on operations, pricing services low, and maintaining an open-door policy for the poor and making little attempt to collect for services, they simply have no reserves for meeting the pressures of the marketplace.

If health care costs were not increasing at high rates and if there were no other pressures on local government, public hospitals might not be in such difficulty. However, many public and community hospitals are in trouble. They are being wooed by national and international companies, large multihospital systems operated by religious and community groups, neighboring hospitals, and a variety of other organizations offering to manage, lease, or buy their operations.

Management Options/Chapter 8
Emerging Strategies

Obviously, not every hospital in the nation is faced with the kind of challenges alluded to in this chapter. Some community and public hospitals enjoy widespread support, have healthy balance sheets, and see opportunities for continued public service. Although chains are growing rapidly and are increasingly becoming the dominant mode of organization in the industry, the existence of innovative, aggressive public and voluntary hospitals offer ample evidence that this traditional approach to delivering health care is not dead.

Some single hospitals have elected to take the lead in developing their own regional system of services. Many have undergone corporate restructuring and established a holding company with for-profit and not-for-profit subsidiaries. Still others have developed local, regional, and national organizations to provide them with the advantages normally offered through large management companies. National organizations, such as the Voluntary Hospitals of America and Hospital Corporation of America, are themselves becoming a resource to their members for developing strong regional relationships, which, in turn, stress the vibrancy of voluntary and public community organizations.

However, some hospital leaders have decided that the road to survival for hospital services in their communities requires the use of outside contract management organizations or the leasing or selling of hospital facilities. Their needs have clearly sent signals to investors, aggressive voluntary hospitals, and a host of other potential suppliers of services. The organizations realize that much of the business of health care can be acquired. They also recognize the profit potential in going after hospitals that can be convinced that it is in their own and their communities' best interests to bring in a new management group. Individual hospital administrators and governing boards may wish it were otherwise. But the growth and development of multihospital systems, the successes they have enjoyed, and the importance of their continued favor in the capital markets make it inevitable that practically every hospital in the nation will at one time or another become a target for acquisition, management, or affiliation. For most hospitals, being considered an acquisition target by another hospital or entity outside the community represents another significant trend in the health care environment.

The foregoing assessment of the current status of the health care field can serve as a starting point for each hospital's analysis of the specific trends that will affect it in the foreseeable future. Such an assessment, along with a hard look at the hospital's strengths and weaknesses within the context of its basic philosophy and mission, should be an integral part of each institution's strategic planning process. After this analysis, a hospital can more precisely decide exactly what the community needs and how its needs can be met.

Decisions about shared services, autonomy, contract management, leases, and sales should be consequences of careful planning and decision making, not responses to crises. Determining community needs after a hospital has been leased

Chapter 8/Management Options

or sold can be an exercise in futility, because the community no longer has the requisite control to make such decisions. Basic planning prior to dealing with the primary issues cited in this chapter is a necessity.

Policy Options

County commissioners, hospital trustees, and other community leaders can contract manage, lease, or sell their hospital. They can also decide to retain the present organizational structure and enhance the management staff and resource base.

Hospitals that decide to remain independent can form consortia to protect their independence and gain economies of scale from certain collective activities. A case in point is the Southeastern Idaho Health Services Consortium. This group of 1 Catholic and 11 county hospitals focuses on strengthening each institution in order to remain independent. So far, the consortium has instituted shared programs in biomedical engineering, quality assurance, utilization review, and in-service education, and it has plans for developing collective expertise in strategic planning and corporate restructuring as well. Another example is the Health Services Consortium run by Virginia Mason Medical Center in Seattle, Washington. This consortium is an organization of 12 urban and rural hospitals working together to expand educational resources, control costs, and improve patient care. These objectives are accomplished through training programs, assistance in strategic planning, and marketing and physician recruitment.

If a hospital board decides to change the organizational arrangements of the hospital, it must consider several perplexing questions:

- Which multihospital system should it choose for affiliation?
- Which system would be best for the community?
- If the hospital chooses an investor-owned system, will the cost of care be higher, because profits are needed for shareholder dividends?
- How will physicians react to a change in the way the hospital conducts business?
- What will happen to the care of indigent patients in the community?
- Will the elderly receive the type of services they need?
- Will the hospital become another unit in a big organization?
- Will the new organization invest new capital in the area?
- Will the governing board continue to direct the hospital, or will another board in another city take on the major governance functions?
- If the hospital enhances its services, will more industry come to the area?
- Will personnel who have families in the community and cannot leave the area be assured of jobs?
- If the hospital affiliates with a large system, how can it be certain that the care the community receives will continue to reflect the hospital's values?

- If the hospital chooses a not-for-profit system, how much of its present autonomy will be retained?

These and other concerns surface when an organizational change of this magnitude is contemplated. The hospital must perform a comprehensive analysis of each organizational arrangement, delineate its advantages and disadvantages, and fully debate the ramifications of each course of action before making a decision. As the final step, broad criteria of organizational excellence should be applied in selecting the multihospital system that will bring about the desired structural changes.

Therefore, two major decisions facing policymakers for small and rural hospitals are:

- Which organizational arrangement is best for the hospital? Should the hospital remain independent? Or should it consider contract management, lease, or sale?
- If the hospital decides not to remain independent, which multihospital system is best for the community?

Independence Option

To remain independent does not mean to retain the status quo. Instead, independence means transforming the present rural hospital facility into a strongly managed hospital that assumes a vital role in a regional health care system.

Strong management means:

- A solid financial program that maximizes reimbursement
- A human resource system that is built on an equitable wage and salary program, relevant training programs, productivity standards, and a strong performance appraisal mechanism
- Management of supplies and equipment so that the best price is paid with no excessive waste and supplies are available when they are needed
- An organized strategic planning and marketing program that highlights the needs of the community and then develops services to meet those needs
- Trustee and physician education that enables hospital leaders to keep abreast of health care changes so they can respond quickly to competitive pressures

Through the strategic planning process, rural hospital leadership determines the strengths and weaknesses of the hospital, the threats to its existence, and the opportunities that are available to it. Strategies that maximize the strengths and minimize weaknesses and threats are developed.

One decision that has to be made is the determination of what the institution will become in the future. If it is better for the community that the hospital

Chapter 8/Management Options

transform itself into a comprehensive primary care center, then the hospital planning process should recommend diversification into outpatient care, ambulatory surgery, health promotion, and home health care. If a decision is made not to pursue ambulatory care and if acute care is not a viable option, then the leadership should consider transforming the hospital into a long-term-care facility or a rehabilitation center.

Because health care in the future will be delivered by networks of physicians and hospitals tied together by insurance programs, it behooves the leadership of rural hospitals to consider affiliation with one or several networks as soon as possible. There are several reasons for this:

- Being a part of a large organization may assure the health care facility and the rural physicians that they will be able to increase patient volume. Some patients may wish to remain close to home for the majority of their care, but others may want to take advantage of the lower prices charged by health maintenance organizations (HMOs) or the discounted rates of preferred provider organizations (PPOs). Affiliating with organizations offering these options may strengthen the hospital's position with the community.
- Establishing strong referral links between rural hospitals and larger providers enables primary care physicians to play a vital part in the patient care treatment and rehabilitation of patients sent from the rural areas to high-technology centers. Specialists at the high-technology centers are beginning to include their colleagues in rural practice in every aspect of the care regimen. Patients are then assured that they will return home as soon as possible.
- The hospital may realize economies of scale through shared services, such as purchasing, management consulting, and financial and marketing advice, and through access to clinical and managerial specialists that would not have been possible otherwise.

One of the major advantages of belonging to a clinical and managerial network is that the services of the hospital are marketed to employers and consumers. This activity can increase the volume of patients for the hospital. The networks can support the hospital through specialized services and increased patient volume. However, they cannot supply capital for diversification and expansion.

Contract Management, Lease, or Sale Options

If a decision is made not to remain independent but to seek affiliation with a larger system, then the trustees, physicians, and administrators have to decide not only the type of organization with which to affiliate but also the type of service to buy from the larger provider.

Management Options/Chapter 8

Types of Organizations

Almost any organization could conceivably enter the market to acquire hospitals. A neighboring hospital might propose consolidation as a route to improved regional services. A local government might take over a failing, but needed, community or religious hospital. These options have long existed and are fairly well understood, if not universally used as appropriate solutions to particular community problems. Therefore, although they represent important possibilities, they are not discussed in this chapter.

For years hospitals have banded together to jointly produce or sell certain services. Several hundred shared services organizations currently offer dozens of management and some clinical services. Public stock companies serve thousands of hospitals by providing or managing everything from housekeeping to sophisticated materials management and information systems. It is difficult to imagine any service or product a hospital might need that could not be supplied by a contract service. In fact, at the extreme, governing boards and administrators could ultimately become prudent buyers who negotiate and manage the myriad contracts and relations that make up the working relationships currently called a hospital.

Today, one of the most significant problems for the single voluntary and public hospital is how to respond appropriately to overtures to join systems, especially those systems that seek to manage, lease, or own the hospitals with which they affiliate. Therefore, trustees and administrators need to be conversant with the three types of buyer organizations (investor-owned, secular not-for-profit, and not-for-profit religious-sponsored); the nature of each type of new arrangement; the issues likely to arise under each arrangement; and some criteria that can be used to assess the arrangements most likely to be proposed.

According to Arthur Andersen & Co., 6 percent of all hospitals were managed by multihospital systems in 1982 and 3 percent were owned, leased, or controlled by the systems. This same source predicts that by 1995, 13 percent of all hospitals will be managed by multihospital systems and 40 percent of all hospitals will be owned, leased, or controlled by the systems.

According to the *Directory of Multihospital Systems, Multistate Alliances, and Networks* (1985), there are 251 multihospital systems. Of this number, 31 are investor owned, 101 are secular not-for-profit organizations, 98 are Catholic, and 21 are run by other religious groups.

Although industry observers often differentiate between systems on the basis of their ownership and profit or not-for-profit (or taxpaying or nontaxpaying) status, careful review of both types of systems shows that neither offers a free lunch. However, the cost of doing business is different for each type of system, and this difference may become relevant in deciding just what kind of system a community prefers.

131

Chapter 8/Management Options

Investor-Owned Systems

The investor-owned multihospital system has experienced rapid growth in the past 10 years. Projections indicate that by 1990 this type of hospital will constitute 19 percent of the total number of hospitals (Arthur Anderson & Co. and American College of Hospital Administrators, 1984, p. 18). This for-profit structure sells its common and other types of equity stock in the marketplace. As with any stockholder-owned firm, its owners are assumed to expect growth, enhancement of stock values, profits, and dividends.

To achieve such growth, investor-owned systems typically reinvest the bulk of their profits in existing or acquired business opportunities. Like other health care organizations, these firms must also have strong support of the physicians and patients who use their hospitals plus widespread public acceptance of their operations. Without such acceptance, the loss of either patient, physician, or community support could damage immediate profits and the ability of that system to acquire business in other markets.

Investor-owned systems offer a variety of services ranging from overall management or lease of a hospital to the provision of selected management services. Hospitals in these systems are managed by a central office, which:

- Provides central policy and management direction
- Standardizes operating systems and procedures
- Negotiates and controls all major financial transactions
- Provides an array of insurance plans to strengthen market shares for their owned and managed facilities

Of course, investor-owned systems vary widely in their approaches to decision making. Some systems operate in a decentralized manner, and some have central management. The choice between decentralization or centralization is ultimately made by each parent firm, not by individual hospitals in the system.

Health policy leaders believe that the investor-owned sector will own 23 percent of all the nation's hospitals within 10 years (Arthur Andersen & Co. and American College of Hospital Administrators, 1984, p. 30). Whatever the ultimate growth figures, this development represents a significant change in the health care industry.

Secular Not-for-Profit Systems

Secular not-for-profit systems are owned and operated as 501(c)(3) tax-exempt organizations. These systems usually have a community governing board that exercises complete control. Profits are typically reinvested in operations or in new health care ventures in the region.

Hospital systems in this category are restructuring their corporations to establish parent holding companies that coordinate for-profit and not-for-profit subsidiary corporations. Thus, the parent company, through its for-profit subsidiary, can work outside the payment and regulatory constraints imposed on not-for-profit hospitals to provide organizational flexibility in responding to new market opportunities.

Although not-for-profit systems do not pay cash dividends to equity holders, they generally expect each hospital that they manage, lease, or own to pay its way. Short-term loans, small subsidies, or low profit margins may be tolerated, but hospitals are expected to be sufficiently profitable to provide a reasonable return on investment.

For the most part, not-for-profit multihospital systems do not have the capital to buy or lease hospitals at great distances from their home base. However, because contract management requires less capital, it is a likely mode of expansion for these systems. In 1984, secular not-for-profit systems had a 19.1 percent share of all managed beds (Johnson, 1985).

Religious-sponsored not-for-profit systems

Religious-sponsored not-for-profit hospital systems function as 501(c)(3) tax-exempt organizations but are controlled by church organizations. Some types of religious systems are the Catholic organizations, managed mostly by religious orders, and organizations affiliated with other religious groups, including Methodists, Baptists, Lutherans, Seventh-Day Adventists, and Jews.

Some religious systems are focusing on the development of regionally integrated health care systems. These regional entities see their mission as the provision of a broad range of acute care and chronic care services to a defined population base. The services provided might include primary and long-term care, rehabilitation, referral, and health promotion services. The Baptist Hospital System in Birmingham, Alabama, is a good example of this organizational form, as is the Methodist Hospital System in Houston, Texas.

Although some regional systems offer services to hospitals outside their immediate regions, most regional systems seem more interested in serving local hospitals. The primary motivation behind regional systems is to build the region's resources to ensure minimal duplication of scarce tertiary clinical and managerial resources. For example, such systems offer clinical services to better utilize resources and to encourage greater affinity among the clinical personnel of all their units. In contrast, national chains attempt sharing of clinical resources by entering into affiliations with regional hospitals. Some firms also offer a number of discrete clinical services to managed and owned hospitals as well as to other independent hospitals. Increasingly, regional systems also offer prepaid plans and preferred provider arrangements.

Services Sold by Multihospital Systems

Multihospital systems offer hospitals definite services or products. The three most important are contract management, lease, and sale.

Chapter 8/Management Options

Contract management, as used in this chapter, means the general day-to-day management of one organization by another under a formal contract. The managing organization reports directly to the governing board or owners of the managed organization, who retain total legal responsibility for and ownership of the facility's assets and liabilities. Such institutional management is distinguished from departmental management, in which the contract management firm and local manager report to the chief executive officer of the hospital.

A *lease* is a contract that provides for the exclusive possession and profits from lands and buildings for life or for a specified period. To lease a hospital is to sell full use and responsibility for the hospital to another party. Thus, the organization holding the lease has complete control over the operation and thrust of the institution.

The *sale* of a hospital means that all rights, assets, buildings, and land are transferred, for consideration, to another party forever. Of course, sales can have conditions attached to them, but basically a sale takes the former owner out of the operation except for any specifically contracted-for conditions.

Contract Management

Contract management of the entire operation has fewer irreversible consequences than either lease or sale. This approach to managing organizations has a long history, and it can work well. The broad range of support it provides to the administrator often enhances management's role in the institution.

The major criticism of contract management revolves around two major issues. First, it is argued that the contract manager cannot bring more to a hospital than can a competent administrator working with a governing board that understands hospital management. There is undoubtedly much truth in this assertion. Granted, many contract management firms offer the expertise of specialists and shared purchasing contracts, but these can also be bought directly from other vendors. Whether one approach is ultimately more cost-effective than another depends on the resources necessary to raise the standards of the hospital. Still, some hospitals have indicated a preference for contract services. They like the way contract management works, and they retain ownership and can negotiate new contracts when the first agreement runs out.

Second, contract management firms have been criticized because they place their interests above those of the hospitals they manage. Some potential for a duality of interest does exist. Conflicts can arise when it comes to weighing the interests of a hospital and those of the management firm. When the hospital's chief executive officer, who is responsible for being the eyes and ears of the hospital and the implementor of hospital policy, is also an employee of the management firm, the potential is greater than if any other level of hospital employee is involved. Trustees may want to consider using an outside audit team to periodically assess the operation of the management contract, just as they do to evaluate financial performance.

Management Options/Chapter 8

This criticism of contract management becomes even more important in light of assertions by contract managers that they often take on contracts in hopes of gaining an opportunity to lease or buy the hospital. Some managers will take on contracts only if they can get an option to buy later or, at least, a right of first refusal should the governing board ultimately decide to sell or lease.

There is no inherent problem with a firm contracting with a hospital in hopes of later acquisition nor with a hospital hiring a management firm and offering it the opportunity to buy if the hospital is consequently put up for sale. However, when the chief executive officer works for both organizations, the potential exists for subtly pushing events toward different outcomes. Again, this is no problem for an alert governing board or other public officials who are keenly cognizant of their fiduciary responsibilities.

A natural question arises in view of those criticisms. Could most hospitals avoid such problems by hiring competent administrators and providing them with good backup resources, access to needed consultants, and shared services? The answer, frequently, is yes. However, many governing boards are equally convinced that they simply cannot be assured that the hospital is on the right course unless they work with a major firm in which all hospital decision makers have confidence. Many governing boards also want to be linked closely to a prestigious national or regional firm with a large staff of management specialists.

Ironically, very small hospitals and those with warring factions (which make management difficult under almost all circumstances) may find that most contract management firms simply will not consider managing them. In addition, hospitals that have exhausted their reasons for existence and should go out of business will have trouble attracting firms to manage their operations. Some firms will recognize these problems for what they are and will not accept contracts to perform an impossible or socially undesirable task. Alternatively, other firms may accept these jobs, but with a clear understanding that the total outcome of their work will likely be the closing of these hospitals and perhaps the building of other needed services for those communities in their stead. Such situations clearly indicate the need for hospitals to do a thorough strategic assessment of their communities and their own needs prior to making other major decisions.

On balance, contract management appears to be a satisfactory service. There are pitfalls to its use, and some hospitals may not be able to secure contract services because of their prospects or internal difficulties that cannot be easily overcome by a management company. A plus is that the existing owners retain policy control and can, with due diligence, direct hospital affairs in much the same manner as they would with their own administrator.

Some firms that offer contract management services also own and lease hospitals. Should a managed hospital later decide to lease or sell, the managing firm becomes a prime candidate for consideration. Because the firm and the hospital

Chapter 8/Management Options

have had opportunities to learn about one another, such transactions seem inevitable.

Organizational buyers with intimate knowledge of the seller's operation have inherent advantages in any bidding process, if indeed any bidding takes place. Because there is a potential for conflict of interest in such proceedings (the hospital's management team works for both the buyer and the seller), the hospital should consider having outside consultants aid in the decision-making process when or if it decides to move from a contract-management situation to a lease or purchase option.

Lease or Sale

The lease or sell options available to hospitals can be looked at together because they have similar characteristics. A lease gives the lessee the right to use the property and all profits from it for a defined period. The lessor is entitled to a payment for such use and may enforce any restrictions agreed to in the lease contract.

A lease can contain virtually any set of conditions that can be agreed to in a bona fide arm's-length transaction between independent parties. If the parties are not independent, then there is a possibility that any dollar transactions between the two might not be considered valid by third-party reimbursement agencies. For instance, if a county or voluntary hospital sets up a separate corporation under its control and that corporation leases the hospital from its original owner and pays a leasing fee, the fee would likely not be treated as a cost of operating the hospital because the lessee and the lessor are commonly controlled, related parties in the transaction. Therefore, this discussion about leasing and selling a hospital assumes an independent transaction. More particularly, it assumes that the buyer is a multihospital system or management company.

A lease contract can, and often does, contain language that requires the lessee to maintain the premises as a hospital (or other health care service), keep certain services in operation (such as emergency departments), and maintain access for the medically indigent. Leases may also require covenants to restrict the hospital's ability to allow abortions or other procedures repugnant to the owners. Of course, a lease is a contract, and one party may impose on the other party only such conditions as that party is willing to accept. If conditions in the lease are likely to become expensive to maintain, for example, a requirement that all indigents be served free, the outside firm may be reluctant to accept them. Care of the medically indigent has created much controversy because of the difficulty in defining it and the concern by lessees that local governments may reduce their contributions to indigent care, thus forcing the lessee to absorb heavy business losses.

Both leasing and sale of the hospital put policy control (bounded only by the explicit terms of the leasing contract or deed) in the hands of a separate, independent organization. In a sale, about the only remaining responsibility of the selling organization is to watch for potential changes that might trigger a reversionary provision in the deed (such as a new owner's attempt to transform the property into a resort hotel when the deed requires that the sold property always be used as a hospital). In a lease, the lessor must pay more attention to the operation because of the number of provisions that require monitoring and the fact that ownership remains with the lessor. The lessor needs to perform certain oversight functions to monitor terms of the lease and ensure that the property and operation are well maintained in case they are returned to the original owner.

Leasing considerations
What a hospital should look for in a lease, as in a management contract, depends to a large extent on its goals in entering the arrangement in the first place. For instance, if the governing board or the political body responsible for running the hospital cannot keep the hospital functioning properly, then leasing or selling the institution to new owners is a possible solution. If, at the same time, the selling or leasing body wants to hold down the cost of institutional services to citizens, then this additional factor becomes a major issue to be considered by the parties.

When the operation is leased rather than sold, the leasing organization must anticipate that at some point, it will need to raise the necessary capital to get back into the hospital business. If it cannot raise the money, it will have no choice but to continue leasing the facility or sell it.

If a hospital's goals are to bring in new ideas, policies, governing board members, management, and directions, can it do so by leasing? The answer is a qualified yes. Because a hospital is an ongoing business and not merely plant and equipment, many existing personnel will continue to work there. Many of the policies in place will remain because they fit the nature and current character of the hospital. Programs will change slowly, because installing new equipment and establishing new procedures and processes take time.

If a local government or community board faces a vexing problem in providing leadership for the institution, leasing the facility to a new organization can provide a good opportunity for change. The lessee can bring in its own management team to serve as the real policy board, enlist different local citizens to advise on policy, or appoint a new local board with policy responsibilities. However, because policy is not made in a vacuum, the local medical staff and its practice patterns, reimbursement rules with their peculiarities, union practices, and the like tend to preclude any major departures from the status quo in the short run.

Without doubt, a new organization has opportunities to avoid the mistakes of the past and to set new directions without much of the rancor that characterizes some hospital boards and political bodies. However, hospitals must remember that solving a leadership problem by turning over the business to another group is a drastic solution and should be considered with great care.

137

Chapter 8/Management Options

Leasing fee

Several questions arise immediately when a hospital considers leasing, and some of these questions center around the leasing fee. For example, what kind of fee should be charged? What will be done with the monies received for the lease? What impact will leasing fees have on the cost of operation and prices paid by consumers? Even more important to most government hospitals, what will happen to indigent care expenditures?

Where does the money paid for a lease or sale go?. Simply put, it goes to the legal owners and can be used in any fashion consistent with their charter of operation. For a local government, that means any governmental function. For a not-for-profit corporation, that means any purpose consistent with its charter and the laws of the state governing such organizations. New foundations funded through such sales have opportunities for serving the poor, meeting new health care needs, and helping in other less well-funded areas of care.

Some governmental officials elect to lease the hospital and put the lease or rental payments in the county treasury for general use, including welfare and health care services for the medically indigent. Some officials place these funds in special accounts to be used to support indigent care. However the funds are used, the cost of these payments to the former operator becomes a cost of the new operator's business. As such, the cost must be recovered by increased efficiencies, increased charges to consumers, or both.

Although such legal uses may seem straightforward, any government or not-for-profit corporation can expect queries, pressures, and other efforts to apply lease or sale proceeds to health care, not highways, sewers, or other less-related activities. Some critics may argue that once a community has invested in health care through taxes and contributions, the proceeds should not be used in other pursuits, even though such uses may be clearly legal. Although these arguments may seem trivial, they should be taken seriously, especially in communities that might want to take over the local hospital after a lease terminates or might be in a position to buy back a sold hospital or put some new health care service into place.

If the hospital is leased for a nominal amount, say a dollar a year, and an agreement is made that the current or some related amount of indigent care be provided without further charges to the county, then the cost of the lessee operation would increase by only the amount of the profit needed to justify being in business in that location. In this type of lease, the cost to consumers would increase only by the amount needed for profits, minus any efficiencies that the new operator brought about.

For example, a county hospital that has a profit (excess of receipts over expenses) of 2 percent per year is leased by an investor-owned firm with an after-tax profit of 6 percent on gross revenues. For the firm to achieve its profit level, the hospital would need to generate a 12 percent gross profit level (federal taxes take 6 percent), or 10 percent more than was considered necessary by the previous owner. Assuming precisely the same scope of operations under both owners, the lease arrangement will increase costs to consumers and add a federal tax burden to local hospital services that did not exist before. As for local taxes, the for-profit firm will contribute to the local tax base through property tax assessments. In turn, all such taxes will be passed to consumers through increased charges and taxes.

If, instead, this same county hospital signs a lease with a not-for-profit firm, the cost increases would be less by the amount of the federal income tax burden that is imposed on the investor-owned company. Thus, to attain a 6 percent net profit, the not-for-profit firm, which pays no income taxes, need only increase earnings by 4 percent of gross revenues. (The 6 percent difference is the federal income tax burden.) Even though not-for-profit firms normally pay no local taxes, some communities require user fees in lieu of taxes.

Control over leasing services

New owners of a hospital typically want to improve old programs and install new ones in order to maximize revenue potential. Much of what a new owner wants to do could, and in many cases should, have been done by the old owners. New and former owners may differ over what they consider are needed changes. In such a situation, a lease may give the right to make that decision to the lessee and not to the former operators, or lessors.

Any new programs will be paid for as they would have been regardless of owner. If the new programs are more elaborate than those that might have been approved by a county government but still meet the test of medical need, then the charges for all parties who use the hospital will be increased. This includes the county's responsibility for indigent care as well.

Once a lease is put into operation, control over programs, which are the major determinant of health care costs to the community and to the political body involved, shifts to private parties and away from the government or community board. The obligation of government and users remains to pay the cost, which includes profits and federal and other taxes, of services that are ordered by physicians on their behalf.

Termination of a lease

An important issue to consider is what happens if and when a lease runs out or if, for some reason, the lessor or lessee chooses to terminate. The easy answer is that the lessor resumes ownership and full control. The ease of such a transition, however, depends primarily on the current financial condition of the lessor. Working capital must be raised. Undepreciated values of equipment and supplies must be paid to the lessee, and the undepreciated costs of capital expansion must be assumed or paid off.

Even if the lessor is a county government, which took payment for its undepreciated values at the time of the lease and banked its lease payments at handsome interest rates, the capital needed to resume control would still probably exceed the dollars saved. This situation occurs because the lessee has probably made substantial improvements and added programs, all of which can increase the operation's revenue potential. If, instead of creating a fund to pay for eventual reentry, the county government or other owner used its revenues to pay for indigent care or some other public service, then reentry costs would begin to compare with those of going into business again. Thus, a long-term lease has many of the same characteristics as outright sale of the facility. Control is gone. After a few years, the capital in the operation belongs to the lessee, not the original owner-operator. Therefore, a decision to lease for a long-term period is tantamount to a sale and should be undertaken with the same deliberate approach as if the owner were deciding to get out of the hospital business entirely.

Sale characteristics
When a property is sold outright, the new owners acquire all rights and responsibilities for its operation. What creates confusion and concern over the sale and disposal of public and private hospitals is the possibility that the new owners will care less about all of the problems formerly solved by the county, city, or voluntary organization, such as indigent care, day care, pregnancy clinics, and the like.

Unless the sales contract specifically stipulates that such programs or contingencies be handled in a certain fashion, it is up to the new owner to decide about nongovernmentally mandated programs. The new owner may or may not be as responsive to community needs as the former owner or, indeed, may be even more responsive. Most owners find that their newly acquired hospitals need repair, upgraded equipment, new personnel, and more and better services.

The new owner will decide whether to offer services that cannot be supported by reimbursement, private pay, or government subsidy at the expense of profits and survival. However, hospitals should not automatically reject national or regional multihospital systems merely because they may not willingly subsidize services that the sellers found difficult to subsidize themselves. Hospitals should instead ask whether or not these systems will devote time and energy to building the community and political support necessary to obtain funds for essential community health services. An investigation of the track records of potential buyers in other communities will provide the answer.

Framework for Decision Making

So far, this analysis has distinguished between contract management, lease, and sale options from the standpoint of control. The treatment of these issues is not meant to be exhaustive. The aim, instead, is to alert hospitals to some fundamental concerns that must be faced.

Choice of an Organizational Arrangement

This chapter has discussed distinctions among three major types of organizational arrangement: contract management, lease, and property sale. As stated earlier, the arrangement that gives the governing board the most latitude as to involvement in hospital operations and determination of its destiny is contract management. With this option, organizational autonomy is assured, and the hospital can take advantage of specialized management expertise and the economies of scale associated with larger hospital systems. At the end of the specified contract period, the board can reevaluate the arrangement and decide to continue it or choose another arrangement.

The lease arrangement provides much less freedom. Once stipulations are specified in the lease agreement and it is signed, the lessee has complete control over the hospital's operation. The present board is no longer necessary. Different management styles, procedures, and systems will be employed, and the philosophy of care of the leasing organization prevails. The community will continue to receive care, but at times, the costs may be higher. No assurance is given about the introduction of new comprehensive services as community needs change. There is no guarantee that the care will be better, worse, or the same. Nor is it certain whether the hospital will collaborate with other health care agencies and hospitals to deliver vertically integrated services. At the end of the lease period, the lessor is free to reclaim the property and the assets at the present value. Sometimes this option is unattainable, especially if there have been substantial capital improvements.

Of the three options, the sale of the hospital is the most final. Through this transaction, all control and responsibility for the delivery of care is transferred to the new owner. With this arrangement, the persons most at risk are the governing board and administrative staff. Other personnel are likely to continue to be employed, and the community will have health services as before.

Before any decision about an organizational arrangement is made, it is advisable to analyze how legal liability and human resource capability differ under each arrangement.

Choice of Multihospital System

Increasingly, small and rural hospital decision makers are faced with an array of organizational vendors selling a variety of services and organizational arrangements. All of them have polished presentations and fancy backup material. They promise a panorama of goods and services and claim that theirs is the most cost-effective. The dilemma faced by most governing boards is how to determine the strengths and weaknesses of each vendor and arrive at a decision that will be best for the community.

Chapter 8/Management Options

Selection criteria based on indicators of excellence can be applied to multihospital systems. These criteria, which reflect the goals of all hospitals throughout the country, are embodied in the following questions:

- How does this organization compare with similar organizations?
- Will this organization help the hospital deliver comprehensive, accessible, continuous, high-quality, and humane health care services?
- Will this organization strengthen the hospital as a service organization, improve its management and human resource capability, and ensure that it meets its local responsibilities?
- Will this organization maximize the hospital's financial resources?

Examining each multihospital system against these criteria and against each other helps to keep the decision-making process objective. Decision makers also have to decide how important each of these criteria is to the hospital at this time.

References

Arthur Andersen & Co. and American College of Hospital Administrators. *Health Care in the 1990s: Trends and Strategies.* Chicago: Arthur Andersen & Co. and ACHA, 1984, pp. 18, 30.

Directory of Multihospital Systems, Multistate Alliances, and Networks. 6th ed. Chicago, IL: American Hospital Publishing, Inc., 1985.

Johnson, Donald. Investor-owned chains continue expansion, 1985 survey shows. *Modern Healthcare.* 1985 June 7. 15(12):75.

Chapter 9

Physician Recruitment

Joe B. Lawley
H. Neil Copelan

The need for primary care physicians in rural areas throughout the United States is well known, and the consensus is that the need can be met, not by increasing the number of physicians generally, but by evening out the geographic distribution of physicians. This solution is simple to state but difficult to achieve. There seems to be no proven method of distributing physicians to areas of need.

Although physician recruitment without regard to the quality of the "marriage" between doctor and community is relatively easy, building and maintaining a high-quality, harmonious medical staff is difficult. When accomplished, however, a synergistic effect permeates the entire community. Public perception of individual physicians and the entire staff is enhanced when local physicians trust one another and refer patients to one another. The converse is also true.

Those who are unfamiliar with or unsuccessful at recruiting physicians to their community may think that persons must be "born" recruiters or professional recruiters to succeed. Although some individuals are indeed more adept at recruiting than are others, a well-planned and well-executed recruitment program can improve results for everyone. No one has a greater interest in the quality and quantity of physicians in a community than its own citizens. Therefore, recruiting can be done more effectively and efficiently by local people than by professional recruiting firms.

This chapter assists hospital administrators in building the optimum medical staff by identifying some of the ingredients necessary for successful, locally originated, cost-effective physician recruitment. These elements, while not exclusive, can be determined at least in part by answering the following questions:

Chapter 9/Physician Recruitment

- What are the factors that influence physicians' decisions about practice locations?
- What are the factors that influence young physicians to leave a rural practice?
- What are the strategies and issues at the state level that will assist physician recruitment in rural communities?
- What are the factors that distinguish communities that are successful in physician recruitment from those that are not?
- What are the successful strategies used by rural hospital administrators to recruit physicians?

Practice Locations

According to the Southern Regional Education Board, the following six factors, listed in order of importance, influence the decisions of physicians concerning their selection of a practice location (McPheeters, 1985):

- Geographic preference (urban or rural, North or South)
- Professional opportunity and challenge
- Family needs and preferences
- Availability of professional peers and facilities
- Potential for adequate income
- Availability of social and recreational opportunities

Factors that influence physicians' decisions about practice locations may change from place to place and from time to time. Therefore, looking at local or statewide studies that have been made on this subject is beneficial. The number-one factor, geographic preference, is quite important. Identifying those residents (both physician and spouse) who have an interest in a rural practice and a life-style that is conducive to rural living is of primary consideration.

One factor that is not specifically mentioned in the study conducted by the Southern Regional Education Board but that greatly influences the location decision of a new physician is the attitude of local physicians. The professional opportunity given the new physician in a rural community is largely determined by the local physicians.

A study on the effect of the factor of adequate income on physician recruitment in rural areas was recently completed by the Small Business Development Center of the University of Georgia (Kenney, 1983). The study indicated that physicians desiring to practice in rural communities of 15,000 population or less believe that the most helpful types of financial assistance, in order of priority, are:

- Rent-free office
- Low-interest loans
- Guaranteed salary

- Interview or moving expense reimbursement
- Free medical equipment

On the other hand, Georgia rural communities are most likely to offer the following, in order of priority (Kenney, 1983):

- Interview or moving expense reimbursement
- Rent-free office
- Guaranteed salary
- Paid utilities
- Paid clerical staff

Physicians and communities are usually not far apart on what physicians believe is needed and what communities provide. However, physicians do believe that low-interest loans and free medical equipment are important.

A guaranteed salary does not, in many cases, mean literally granting a lump sum of money to the new physician. It simply means that the new physician can count on that salary figure. If he or she does not reach that income figure during the first year of practice, the community guarantees that it will make up the difference between the actual income and the guaranteed income.

The community should decide what inducements, such as moving expenses, guaranteed salary, rent-free office space, and paid utilities and clerical staff, it will offer to prospective physicians. Moving expenses require a one-time payment, but this is not true of the other benefits mentioned. Therefore, the community must specify how long it intends to supply these benefits. It should not be supplying these benefits indefinitely.

Leaving Rural Practice

A study of the practice problems of rural physicians in communities of fewer than 10,000 population in Georgia (Brown, 1985) found that the following seven factors affect rural physicians three times more than urban physicians:

- Adequacy of hospital facilities
- Availability of professional colleagues and associates
- Opportunities for professional education
- Isolation
- Emergency department coverage
- Personalities and practice style of physicians in the local community
- Cultural activities

The study pointed out that "the single largest resource for the physician making the transition from training to practice is an established physician in the community where he chooses to practice" (Brown, 1985). One of the most important pieces of information a community can obtain is to find out why a physician decides to leave a rural practice. The community should also try to find out why a physician who showed an interest in the community decided not to practice there.

Once a physician is recruited, the job is only half completed. Considerable effort and attention need to be given to retaining the new physician.

In most states, there are resources available to identify in-state residents who are interested in a primary care practice. A community should seek out these resources for leads to physicians who are seeking a rural practice location.

State-Level Strategies and Issues

Strategies at the state level to assist in physician recruitment include the funding of primary care residency programs, particularly family practice residencies to augment the supply of physicians in the state and especially in rural areas of the state. Some states have special admission requirements stipulating that a certain number of students entering medical school be residents of the state and have a rural background. Many states have loan forgiveness and scholarship programs that grant state funds to students on the condition that they serve for a specified number of years in a rural community or in an area that has a shortage of physicians. Other state-level actions that influence the distribution of physicians include the following (McPheeters, 1985):

- Recruiting medical students with experience or high desire to work in settings or specialties where professionals are needed
- Giving these students loans or work-study contracts that are forgiven for service in needed areas but that require severe penalties for defaults
- Providing strong academic instruction about practice in needed specialties and settings
- Providing clinical training in needed specialties and settings
- Providing residency training in needed specialties and settings
- Offering role models and counseling for practice in needed settings
- Having communities recruit and assist needed professionals in locating in these settings
- Ensuring reasonable income for work in needed areas
- Modifying laws and regulations to allow practitioners to practice as effectively as possible

A combination of the above actions and other strategies to influence the decisions of physicians to practice in rural areas is necessary in order to ensure success. One example of an attempt to combine some of these strategies resulted in what is called the Georgia Medical Fair. This program is a cooperative effort of seven agencies to plan and provide a physician recruitment conference, or medical fair. The purpose of the fair, which is held each year in the fall, is to allow medical students, residents, and representatives from communities that have a population of 15,000 or less and that have a hospital to discuss practice opportunities in the state. The seven private and public agencies presently sponsoring the fair include the State Medical Education Board, Medical Association of Georgia, Medical College of Georgia, Georgia Academy of Family Physicians, Georgia Hospital Association, Joint Board of Family Practice, and University of Georgia Cooperative Extension Service.

Working together, designated staff from these agencies use the medical fair as a program mechanism to develop and provide coordinated information and organizational services to both rural communities and medical residents to influence and enhance effective contacts and practice arrangements. The results of the medical fairs held from 1979 to 1983 have been the direct placement of 83 residents in Georgia communities of 15,000 population or less or with the Georgia Department of Human Resources.

The medical fair concept, which began in 1979, is no longer considered an experiment. An increasingly proven method of combating the maldistribution of physician services in Georgia, the medical fair is unique in several respects:

- Voluntary agency coordination: Seven private and public health-related agencies share their resources to efficiently and effectively place physicians in the nonurban areas of Georgia.
- Orientation for participants: A special meeting is held each year for community representatives planning to attend the medical fair. At this meeting, community marketing strategies are discussed, and current research on rural physician recruitment and retention is shared. Likewise, resident physicians are briefed before the fair on how to select a community and set up a practice.

The medical fair is one example of what coordinated strategies can do. Another statewide service might be a central information system that rural community representatives seeking a physician could use at a central location to secure desired information on all physicians in residency programs in the state. Another useful service would be a state-supported agency that would provide consultant service at no or minimum charge to the rural community to assist it in organizing its recruitment effort. If these or other services are not provided, rural hospital administrators and other groups, such as the Chamber of Commerce, locally elected state representatives, local physicians, Farm Bureau, and municipal league, might join together in requesting these services from appropriate state and private agencies.

The one important issue at the state level in Georgia at the present time is whether an agency or agencies in the health care field should focus solely on the placement of physicians primarily in medically underserved rural areas or focus simultaneously on the placement of physicians in both medically underserved rural and urban areas. Rural communities must request that priority attention and assistance be given to their medical needs. This focused assistance might come from one agency or from several agencies in cooperation. If no priority is given to rural areas, then those rural communities with the greatest need might not receive enough assistance. The problem of maldistribution deserves an organized priority to influence physicians to locate in rural areas.

Communities Successful in Recruitment

To attract a physician to a community is to attract a small industry, and the community must approach this problem as a total community concern. The leadership of the community must first agree that a physician is needed and then decide on a marketing plan to attract this new industry. In particular, three key leaders within the community must be positive about the marketing plan and participate in it. They are the local hospital administrator, local physicians, and the local banker. "The smaller a community is, the more it needs to develop a leadership group to provide assistance, advice, and moral support to the health professionals that have been recruited" (Bruce, 1985).

McConnell, Kohls, and Norton (1984) tried to determine what made one community so much more attractive than another to physicians who wanted a small-town practice. One community characteristic stood out: the successful rural community was one that was perceived by its own community representatives as being a town that had the ability to confront problems and take necessary action. The community must be able to "get its act together." This simple statement is critical to a community's ability to attract and retain a physician.

Successful Strategies*

Long-Range Planning Committee

The recruitment process essentially begins with the long-range planning committee, which determines just what services the hospital can afford to provide.

---

*This section is written from the perspective of the administrator of a 70-bed hospital in a rural community (12,000 persons in the city, 30,000 plus in the market area). Four other small hospitals are located 9 to 30 miles away, and major medical centers are 40 and 60 miles away. Approximately 13 percent of the population is more than 65 years old. Per capita income is only slightly higher than the federal poverty level (28 percent of the total population is below the poverty level). The community is a mixture of light industry and agriculture, with agriculture being dominant. The population is generally poor and relatively uneducated (9 percent of the citizens over 25 years old have four or more years of college). The hospital authority is moderately active but clearly expects the administrator to lead the hospital in the appropriate direction. The hospital is a 33-year-old Hill-Burton facility with a history of high administrator turnover and a reputation for mediocre care.

Under the prospective pricing system, with its use of diagnosis-related groups as the key to payment, rural hospitals may no longer be able to provide a complete spectrum of services. They may have to concentrate on those services that they can provide most effectively and efficiently.

The long-range planning committee may use a formal market research study or rely solely on the opinions of committee members (or a combination of these techniques) to identify what additional physician and hospital services are needed. These services should be listed in order of priority and compared to existing capabilities. Such a comparison indicates what kind of and how many specialists are needed. The required specialities should be listed in order of priority to ensure that the community's needs are met adequately. Potential medical staff vacancies caused by physicians' discontinuing their practices must be included in recruiting plans.

The long-range planning committee presents its findings to the governing board. If, on the basis of these findings, the governing board decides that its mission is not being fulfilled because of inadequate quality, quantity, or mix of specialists, it should make the decision to begin the recruitment of needed physicians. After the recruitment decision has been made, the governing board develops and approves a recruitment timetable that is compatible with budget projections.

Recruiting Team

The governing board selects who will serve on the recruiting team and who will be the team leader. Because physician recruitment is so time-consuming, the membership of the recruiting team and the long-range planning committee should be different, although one or two persons might be members of both groups. Also, the recruiting team should be conceived as an ad hoc and not a permanent committee of the hospital. It is the recruiting team's job to actually do the recruiting. Once the physician has come to and is established in the community, the recruiting team can be disbanded. The long-range planning committee, on the other hand, may be a permanent part of the hospital's structure (see chapter 5).

The recruiting team should not be too large. Ideally, it should consist of from seven to nine members. To be effective, team membership should include persons from hospital management, the medical staff, the governing body, and the community. Typically, an executive from the Chamber of Commerce and a local banker participate.

Each team member has specific assignments. For example, the hospital administrator may develop a prospect list, make contact with the physicians, and coordinate interviews and visits. Governing body members should be available to discuss hospital history, philosophy, and future plans. The executive from the Chamber of Commerce may conduct a tour of the area and serve as a resource

Chapter 9/Physician Recruitment

person regarding demographics and industry plans. Medical staff members may be asked to have breakfast with the prospective physician and give him or her a tour of the hospital. If appropriate, the staff doctors may organize an informal social gathering at a physician's home so that the prospect and spouse can meet other local physicians and spouses.

Team Leader

A leader for the recruiting team should be appointed by the governing body to coordinate the entire recruitment effort. Generally, the team leader is the hospital administrator, although other individuals may be acceptable.

The person given the recruiting responsibility must ensure that persons in authority are available to prospective physicians. It is important that prospects know that recruiting them is a high priority for the hospital, medical community, and other citizens.

The team leader must also know how much authority he or she has to make commitments at appropriate times. Without this authority, the "moment" might be lost and, along with it, the prospect. The team leader should also be aware of what kind and how much financial assistance the hospital is willing to make available.

Recruitment Plan

To be consistently successful in recruiting, the hospital must have a well-constructed, detailed recruitment plan. Used often and fine-tuned through experience, the plan can be valid for many years, even with different participants. A sound, well-rehearsed plan is the basis for professional recruiters' successes and is no less appropriate for local community people. A good plan, combined with genuine community interest, can cause the recruitment effort to be extraordinarily successful, especially regarding the physician's compatibility with the community.

Successful implementation of the recruiting plan requires careful education of team members. Each team member should have the freedom to demonstrate his or her personality, express opinions, and interact comfortably and naturally with prospective physicians. Having one or more orientation sessions with the team members develops a level of common understanding. Such a consensus may prevent contradictions, which could arise as the prospective physician talks with various members of the team.

Compatibility

One important person in the recruitment process who must not be overlooked is the spouse of the prospective physician. For married physicians, the happiness of the spouse is a major concern. In many instances, the unhappiness of the family can cause physician dissatisfaction. Therefore, the recruiting team must make every effort to ensure that the move to the community is agreeable to the spouse as well as the physician. One way to handle this situation is to have one or more personable and articulate physicians' spouses meet the prospective physician's spouse. Spouse-to-spouse conversations can be an important determinant in successful recruiting.

The importance of compatibility between the prospective physician and the community is undeniable. Therefore, the recruiting team should identify the characteristics desirable in a prospective physician and rank these characteristics according to priority. By identifying characteristics that would be most important to the local patient population, the team's chances of recruiting successfully are greatly enhanced. Similarly, characteristics of a community that are important to prospective physicians should be addressed to prepare the team to talk on these subjects. How the hospital and community can satisfy each prospect's needs must be part of the presentation to prospective physicians.

Routine of Activity

After the team leader and team members have been selected and the characteristics desired in a prospective physician have been identified, a general routine of activity should be determined:

- Obtain information on a large number of physician prospects. Sources may include state scholarship boards, residency program directors, National Health Service Corps, societies of various medical specialties, and local physicians' acquaintances.
- Build a prospect file. A 5 x 8 file card works nicely. For an example of the information that should be put on the card, see figure 9-1, next page.
- Contact prospects according to established priority and criteria. Refine prospect file.
- Check references on those prospects who show promise.
- Meet the primary prospects.
- Arrange a site visit for the prospective physician and spouse.
- Obtain commitment from prospect.
- Follow up and continue communication with prospect.
- Assist the physician in beginning his or her practice in local community.
- Support the physician after he or she begins practice.
- Fulfill any financial commitments.

Community and Staff Salespersons

The team leader can multiply the chances for successful recruiting by enlisting the aid of as many "salespersons" as possible. Every community has individuals

Chapter 9/Physician Recruitment

Figure 9-1. Information Included on Index Card for Each Candidate

Physician's Name: _____ Specialty: _____

Address: _____ Date Available: _____

Phone Numbers: _____

Education:

College:

Medical School:

Residency:

Personal Data (spouse's name, children, physician's birthday, hometown, etc.):

Record of Activity:

Date	Type of Contact	Comments

who promote a positive image of the area. These salespersons may be from all walks of life. Local physicians can be invaluable salespersons. By communicating the plans and the need for recruiting to the medical staff, the team can learn who supports the plan and who does not. Physicians supportive of the plans can be asked to become active participants in the recruiting effort. The team must also determine the appropriate behavior for handling physicians who are hostile to the plan.

Sometimes the local physician may object to the hospital's decision to recruit additional physicians. However, once the hospital has determined that recruiting another doctor will benefit the community, the hospital should proceed despite any resistance. The local physician will generally decide to cooperate, but if not, the prospective physician should be informed of the local doctor's resistance. Under no circumstances should a local physician's resistance be allowed to divert, stall, or stop the recruitment process.

The hospital's employees can also be salespersons, and therefore memos and department meetings should be used to make all employees aware of the recruiting activity. The hospital's employees should be prepared to respond to questions from prospective physicians who tour the facility during site visits. The team also needs to communicate its plans to the governing body.

Educating the community enhances the chances for successful recruiting. By word of mouth, media attention, and appearances at civic clubs, the recruiting team can stimulate the whole community regarding the importance of attracting physicians. This mass communication effort can also increase the community's interest in the hospital and consequently can provide an excellent opportunity to build a positive image of the hospital. The recruiting team should make as many persons aware of physician recruitment as possible so that prospective physicians who visit the area sense that the entire community wants them.

A word of caution on including too many persons in the recruitment effort too soon. The community may become disappointed and discouraged if they get excited about a prospective physician who subsequently decides not to settle in the community. Therefore, the team leader must exercise good judgment regarding the timing of involving community people other than those who are on the recruiting team.

Importance of Trust

Specific concerns of prospective physicians are identified at the beginning of this chapter. Each team develops its own "packages" to be offered to physicians to satisfy these concerns or needs.

Overriding these tangible items, however, is an intangible that will cause physicians to commit to a community even when the "package" is not what the physicians wanted or, conversely, to reject a community that promised everything they asked for. This intangible is the development of a good rapport and feeling of trust between prospective physician and recruiting team. If trust is established, the prospect will have confidence in the community and in those with whom he or she will work. In addition, the prospect's concern regarding the myriad unknown possible situations that may occur will be diminished. The team can communicate trustworthiness by being conscious of the following points:

- Communicate that the prospective physician is special to the community and that the community really wants him or her
- Display the personality of the community. Let the prospective physician get to know the community, "warts and all." After all, if the community successfully hides its blemishes until after the physician has made a life-changing commitment, the likelihood of a good, long-term relationship with the community, the hospital, and fellow physicians is jeopardized, and a disagreeable situation is likely to develop.
- Be honest. It is unlikely that the community will offer a utopian situation. Everyone must make choices. Although there may be areas of concern to the physician that cannot be eliminated, overall positiveness and trust frequently outweigh objections. It is imperative that the physician be aware of the good and the bad so that decisions are made on the basis of accurate information to minimize the possibility of later unhappiness for everyone.

Conclusion

By involving various people in the recruiting effort, the recruiting team can develop a strong bond between community leaders, hospital staff, physicians, and governing body members. Successful recruiting benefits the community not only medically but also financially (physician families are consumers), socially (physician families frequently make a positive impact through interaction with other townspeople), and civically (physicians and spouses are often asked to participate in local organizations).

Participation by various citizens allows them to take pride in their particular contribution to a successful recruitment. The team should carefully select candidates to be invited for a site visit so that there are a minimum of such visits. The excitement, pleasure, and satisfaction experienced by the participants in a physician site visit will diminish unless doctors are successfully recruited. Therefore, the team should cultivate the prospect, have a sense of the probability of obtaining a commitment during or after the site visit, and generally cause the site visit to be the climax of the recruiting effort. At the close of this stage of the recruiting plan, the team leader, after reviewing all the activity and the assistance available to the prospective physician, should ask for a commitment. The team may do everything correctly to recruit physicians and yet fail simply because the prospects were never actually asked or expected to commit to the community.

A final point to be emphasized is that professional recruiting firms cannot compete with a local recruiting team. Although the professionals may have a large number of prospects, they cannot communicate the virtues of a practice opportunity and the personal satisfaction of living in the community with the same credibility as the local people can. A well-planned, well-executed local recruiting effort is not only cost-effective compared to commercial recruiting, but it is also unparalleled in yielding quality physician-community combinations.

References

Brown, E. Evan, and others. *A Comparison of Beginning Practice Problems Encountered by Rural and Urban Physicians.* Research report 477. Athens, GA: Agricultural Experiment Station, University of Georgia, 1985.

Bruce, Thomas A. Physicians. In: Rural practice: how do we prepare providers. *Journal of Rural Health.* 1985 Jan. 1(1):18.

Kenney, Sandra. *Physician Recruitment to Rural Georgia Communities.* Athens, GA: Small Business Development Center, Institute for Business, University of Georgia, 1983 (CBES monograph 84-101).

McConnell, Diane C., Kohls, James M., and Norton, Richard W. Factors influencing recruitment and retention in two types of rural communities. In: *Improving Rural Health.* Little Rock, AK: Rose Publishing Company, 1984.

McPheeters, Harold L. Influencing the distribution of physicians and other health professionals. *Issues in Higher Education.* Issue 21. Atlanta, GA: Southern Regional Education Board, 1985.

Bibliography

This bibliography was selected and compiled by the Library of the American Hospital Association, a component of the AHA Resource Center, at the request of the Section for Small or Rural Hospitals.

General

Arnold, A. *The Utilization of Quantitative Techniques in Staffing a 49-Bed Rural Hospital.* Chicago: Center for Hospital Management Engineering, American Hospital Association, 1980.

Chen, M. K. Health care services and health status in a rural setting: the utility of some predictors. *Inquiry.* 1982 Fall. 19(3):257-61.

Christianson, J. B., and Faulkner, L. The contribution of rural hospitals to local economies. *Inquiry.* 1981 Spring. 18(1):46-60.

Couto, R. A. Vein dreams: rural health care in a troubled economy. *Health PAC Bulletin.* 1984 Mar.-Apr. 15(2):17-19.

Fiedler, J. L. A review of the literature on access and utilization of medical care with special emphasis on rural primary care. *Social Science and Medicine.* 1981 Sept. 15(3):129-42.

Hagebak, B. R. Nail-keg sittin': a rural key to urban interagency coordination. *New England Journal of Human Services.* 1982 Fall. 2(4):14-21.

Hale, P. L., Immel, T., and Moher, S. Is AHCCCS working in the rural areas? *Arizona Medicine.* 1984 July. 41(7):454-58.

Bibliography

Howard, M. E., and Packard, J. Layoffs hit small, rural hospital. *Michigan Hospital.* 1985 Jan. 21(1):17-19.

Kennedy, V. C. Locational aspects of medical care-seeking in a rural population, with some implications for public policy research. *Journal of Health Politics, Policy and Law.* 1980 Spring. 5(1):142-51.

Lapp, R. J. An approach to rural health care delivery. *Nebraska Medical Journal.* 1980 Apr. 65(4):81-82.

Madison, D. L. Role of state and local government in relation to personal health services: a view of rural health services. *American Journal of Public Health.* 1981 Jan. 71(1 Suppl.):89-90.

Management of Rural Primary Care. Chicago: Hospital Research and Educational Trust, 1982.

Miller, F., Jr. Bringing medical care to underserved and boosting patient occupancy rate. *Southern Hospitals.* 1980 Sept.-Oct. 48(5):17-18.

Miners, L. A. The family's demand for health: evidence from a rural community. *Advances in Health Economics and Health Services Research.* 1981. 2:85-142.

Moscovice, I. S., and Rosenblatt, R. A. Rural health care delivery amidst federal retrenchment: lessons from the Robert Wood Johnson Foundation's Rural Practice Project. *American Journal of Public Health.* 1982 Dec. 72(12):1380-85.

_____. *The Viability of the Rural Hospital.* Washington, DC: U.S. Government Printing Office, 1982.

Murrin, K. L. Rural hospitals can benefit by aiding centers. *Hospitals.* 1980 Oct. 1. 54(19):75-78.

Oboler, S. K., Blieden, M.A., and others. A mobile internal medicine clinic. *Archives of Internal Medicine.* 1983 Jan. 143(1):97-99.

Pediatric medical center helps to overcome the problems of inadequate health care delivery in a rural area. *Hospitals.* 1982 Feb. 16. 56(4):118-19.

Powers, J. S. Primary care in an underserved area. The Goodlark experience in Middle Tennessee. *Public Health Reports.* 1983 July-Aug. 98(4):390-96.

Reid, R. A., and Smith, H. L. Experience of the Checkerboard Area Health System in planning for rural health care. *Public Health Reports.* 1982 Mar.-Apr. 97(2):156-64.

Reilly, B. J., Legge, J. S., Jr., and Reilly, M. S. A rural health perspective: principles for rural health policy. *Inquiry.* 1980 summer. 17(2):120-27.

Rosenblatt, R. A. *Rural Health Care.* New York City: Wiley, 1982.

Bibliography

Samuels, M. E. Meeting the health needs of rural America: the Kirksville Mission. *Osteopathic Hospitals.* 1980 Mar. 24(3):8-11.

Sheps, C. G., and Bachar, M. Rural areas and personal health services: current strategies. *American Journal of Public Health.* 1981 Jan. 71(1 Suppl.):71-82.

Van Hook, R. T. The evolution of rural hospitals. *Business and Health.* 1985 May. 2(6):32-36.

Wallack, S. *Rural Medicine.* Lexington, MA: D. C. Health and Company, 1981.

Wright, D. D., Kane, R. L., and others. Predicting rural health care utilization with archival data. *Journal of Community Health.* 1982 Summer. 7(4):284-91.

Zetzman, M. R., Heartwell, S. F., and Stefanw, C. Patterns of medical services utilization and health care attitudes in a rural Texas population. *Texas Medicine.* 1980 Jan. 76(1):64-69.

Ambulatory Care

Ashby, J. L., Jr. Management and community factors affecting the financial viability of rural health initiative sites. *Journal of Ambulatory Care Management.* 1981 Nov. 4(4):1-14.

Chaska, N. L., Krishan, I., and others. Use of medical services and satisfaction with ambulatory care among a rural Minnesota population. *Public Health Reports.* 1980 Jan.-Feb. 95(1):44-52.

Fitts, A., III. Good Samaritan Hospital and Nursing Home, Inc., Selma, AL.: hospital affiliated clinics meet health needs of rural poor. *Hospital Progress.* 1981 Feb. 62(2):40-41, 62.

Kleinman, J. C., and Makuc, D. Travel for ambulatory medical care. *Medical Care.* 1983 May. 21(5):543-57.

Reid, R. A., and Smith, H. L. Integrated rural health care systems: managerial implications for design and implementation. *Journal of Ambulatory Care Management.* 1984 May. 7(2):13-28.

Stone, S. Rural health clinics: what has happened; what is to come. *Forum on Medicine.* 1980 Nov. 3(11):712-17.

Auxiliary

Bailey, B. Planning the small hospital gift shop. *Hospital Gift Shop Management.* 1984 Mar. 2(3):43-44, 47-48.

Bibliography

McLarty, G., and Cheshier, B. The auxiliary in the smaller hospital: volunteers can augment small staffs and be valuable liaisons. *Texas Hospitals.* 1981 Oct. 37(5):40-41.

Marvel, H. Does small hospital equal small auxiliary? *Michigan Hospitals.* 1980 Feb. 16(2):25.

Diversification

Friedman, E. Diversifying a rural hospital: a lot of work — and very rewarding. *Trustee.* 1981 Mar. 34(3):17-18, 20-21.

_____. Little hospital has big ideas. *Hospitals.* 1980 Nov. 16. 54(22):89-90, 94.

Golda, E. A. Diversification: a survival strategy for rural hospitals. *Health Care Planning and Marketing.* 1981 July. 1(2):1-10.

Keith, J. M. Satellite hospital: innovation in rural health care. *Hospital Progress.* 1980 Mar. 61(3):34.

Kuntz, E. F. Alternative services: rural hospitals adding services to become healthcare centers. *Modern Healthcare.* 1984 Sept. 14(12):159-60.

Trotzky, E. A partnership for rural healthcare. *Health Services Manager.* 1980 Aug. 13(8):1-3.

Elderly

Barber, H., and others. Helping the rural elderly. *Journal of Gerontological Nursing.* 1984 March. 10(3):105-9.

Haemmerlie, F. M., and Montgomery, R. L. The homemaker needs of the rural frail elderly from a client versus agency perspective. *Home Health Care Services Quarterly.* 1984 Spring. 5(1):61-73.

Jinks, M. J. Reaching the rural elderly through the Council on Aging network. *American Journal of Hospital Pharmacy.* 1981 Nov. 38(11):1778-79.

Palmore, E. Health care needs of the rural elderly. *International Journal of Aging and Human Development.* 1983-84. 18(1):39-45.

Reichel, W. Care of the elderly in rural America. *Maryland State Medical Journal.* 1980 May. 29(5):76-79.

Young, C. L., and others. Organizations as volunteers for the rural frail elderly. *Journal of Volunteer Administration.* 1983 Fall. 2(1):33-44.

Emergency Medical Services (EMS)

Andrews, M. Two rural hospitals respond to ambulance needs. *Michigan Hospitals.* 1980 Jan. 16(1):24.

Bibliography

Bassuk, E. L., Pierce, J. E., and Blanch, A. K. Development of a rural behavioral emergency training program: the Vermont experience. *Community Mental Health Journal.* 1984 Winter. 20(4):313-17.

Basu, R. Use of emergency room facilities in a rural area: a spatial analysis. *Social Science and Medicine.* 1982. 16(1):75-84.

Burge, C. D. Experimental use of mobile satellite communications technology in rural EMS systems. *Emergency Medical Services.* 1980 July-Aug. 9(4):50-51.

Cherry, A., and Pollard, J. Sources of funding for EMS in rural settings. *Emergency Medical Services.* 1980 Nov.-Dec. 9(6):131-32.

Edwards, C. Quality assessment in the emergency room of a small, rural hospital. *Quality Review Bulletin.* 1984 Apr. 10(4):119-23.

Gilmore, K. M., Clemmer, T.P., and others. Commitment to trauma in a low population density area. *Journal of Trauma.* 1981 Oct. 21(10):883-88.

Higgins, D., and Goss, J. R. Jump crews: an approach to rural emergency care. *EMT Journal.* 1980 June. 4(2):29-31.

Johnson, N. J. A first response system, rural style. *Journal of Emergency Medical Services.* 1983 Aug. 8(8):38-40.

Kay, B. J., and Myrick, J. A. An evolution of program implementation strategies for a rural first-responder system. *Journal of Community Health.* 1982 Winter. 8(2):57-68.

Koff, S. Z. Emergency medical services in a rural setting: attitudes of policymakers and consumers. *Journal of Health and Human Resources Administration.* 1981 Summer. 4(1):92-115.

McGlown, K. J. FLATIRON: a MAST service for rural Alabama. *Journal of Emergency Medical Services.* 1983 Nov. 8(11):40-42.

Miller, M. The rural emergency nursing curriculum. *Journal of Emergency Medical Services,* 1980 Apr. 5(2):44-47.

Mucha, P., Jr., Farnell, M. B., and others. A rural regional trauma center. *Journal of Trauma.* 1983 Apr. 23(4):337-40.

Murray, J. Levels of training for a rural state. *Emergency Medical Services.* 1980 Mar.-Apr. 9(2):49-50.

Myrick, J. A., Kay, B. J., and others. Acceptance of a volunteer first-responder system in rural communities: a field experience. *Medical Care.* 1983 Apr. 21(4):389-99.

Newkirk, W. Rural emergency department coverage: comparison of a physician assistant to rotating medical staff members. *Journal of the Maine Medical Association.* 1980 Dec. 71(12):375-77.

Bibliography

Peirce, J. C. Established rural health systems. *EMT Journal.* 1981 Feb. 5(1):40-41.

Podgorny, G. Emergency physician assistants: an important adjunct. *Annals of Emergency Medicine.* 1980 Feb. 9(2):109.

Riner, R. M. Developing medical control in a rural EMS system. *Emergency Medical Services.* 1981 Mar.-Apr. 10(2):22-28.

Rural EMS problems. *EMT Journal.* 1980 Mar. 4(1):78.

Russell, G. Providing emergency services in the small or rural hospital. *Texas Hospitals.* 1980 Oct. 36(5):58-60.

Skiendzielewski, J. J., and Dula, D. J. The rural interhospital disaster plan: some new solutions to old problems. *Journal of Trauma.* 1982 Aug. 22(8)694-97.

Spoor, J. E. Rural advanced EMT training: part III. *Emergency Medical Services.* 1981 Jan.-Feb. 10(1):52-55.

Stricklin, R. O. The rural ED nurse: an expanded role. *Journal of Emergency Nursing.* 1980 Sept.-Oct. 6(5):54-56.

Sytkowski, P. A., Pozen, M. W., and others. An analytic method for the evaluation of rural emergency medical service development. *Medical Care.* 1981 May. 19(5):526-46.

Sytkowski, P. A., D'Agostino, R. B., and others. Testing a model that evaluates options for rural emergency medical services department. *Medical Care.* 1984 Mar. 22(3):202-15.

Thompson, W. B. "Life Flight" brings emergency care to rural mountainous areas. *Hospitals.* 1981 Oct. 1. 55(19):49.

Tye, J., Vargish, T., and others. The role of a hospital-based emergency helicopter service in a rural state. *Emergency Medical Services.* 1980 July-Aug. 9(4):17-20.

Zuschlag, R. Building a rural "dream system." *Emergency Medical Services.* 1981 July-Aug. 10(4):15-17.

Governing Boards

Berger, S. Trustee talent aids small hospital staff. *Modern Healthcare.* 1984 Sept. 14(12):174.

Lennie, J. A. Self-help for rural managers and trustees. *Hospital Forum.* 1981 July-Aug. 24(4):56.

Trustee development program: physician recruitment in small and rural hospitals. *Trustee.* 1980 May. 33(5):17-20.

Health Centers and Clinics

Banahan, B. F., III, and Sharpe, T. R. Evaluation of the use of rural health clinics: knowledge, attitudes, and behaviors of consumers. *Public Health Reports.* 1982 May-June. 97(3):261-68.

Douglas, V. T. Rural health clinics serve "invisible poor." *Forum.* 1980 Aug. 4(3):23-28.

Mechanic, D., Greenley, J. R., and others. A model of rural health care: consumer response among users of the Marshfield Clinic. *Medical Care.* 1980 June. 18(6):597-608.

Reid, R. A., Bartlett, E. E., and Kozoll, R. Implementation of the health center concept in a rural community: a case study. *Journal of Community Health.* 1981 Fall. 7(1):57-66.

Ricketts, T. C., Guild, P. A., and others. An evaluation of subsidized rural primary care programs: III. stress and survival, 1981-82. *American Journal of Public Health.* 1984 Aug. 74(8):816-19.

Ricketts, T. C., Konrad, T. R., and Wagner, E. H. An evaluation of subsidized rural primary care programs: II. The environmental contexts. *American Journal of Public Health.* 1983 Apr. 73(4):406-13.

Sheps, C. G., and others. An evaluation of subsidized rural primary care programs: I. A typology of practice organizations. *American Journal of Public Health.* 1983 Jan. 73(1):38-49.

Health Education Promotion

Hanson, P., Matheson, G., and Reed, P. A. A tri-county needs assessment for the purpose of rural health promotion program development. *Home Healthcare Nurse.* 1983 Sept.-Oct. 1(1):22-26, 28.

Irish, E. M., and Taylor, J. M. A course in self-care for rural residents. *Nursing Outlook.* 1980 July. 28(7):421-23.

Lynch, J. M., and Cochran, S. C. Health promotion package developed for rural communities. *Hospitals.* 1983 July 16. 57(14):62-63.

Outreach program serves rural hospitals, businesses. *Hospital Progress.* 1982 Oct. 63(10):28-29.

Strawhecker, P. Health care system tests videotex in rural America. *Fund Raising Management.* 1983 Oct. 14(8):26, 30, 49.

Sullivan, M. E. A patient education system for a rural primary case centre. *International Journal of Health Education.* 1981. 24(2):113-17.

Bibliography

Health Manpower

Antes, E. J. The rural area hospital can afford a librarian. *Bulletin of the Medical Library Association.* 1982 Apr. 70(2):233-36.

Baker, S. A. Rural hospitals' lab workers feel they need more training. *Modern Healthcare.* 1984 Sept. 14(12):178.

Boissoneau, R. Education needs of rural hospital administrators in Arizona. *Hospital and Health Services Administration.* 1982 Mar.-Apr. 27(2):72-78.

───── . The need for professional administrators in rural hospitals. *Hospital and Health Services Administration.* 1984 Mar.-Apr. 29(2):46-55.

Boissoneau, R., Dolan, T., and others. Factors influencing student selection of rural health service administration. *Hospital and Health Services Administration.* 1981. 26(Special Issue 1):48-62.

Duelm, L. C. Medical records consultants: valued members of the small hospital team. *Texas Hospitals.* 1980 June. 36(1):22-23.

Flower, J. Profile of a rural hospital administrator: Vitek's week. *Hospital Forum.* 1983 Sept.-Oct. 26(5):7-12.

Lugenbeel, A. G. Rural-trained technicians stay rural. *Hospitals.* 1980 Sept. 1. 54(17):74-75.

May, P. T., Rosenweig, R., and Liebhaber, L. Circuit rider librarian provides services to small hospitals. *Hospital Progress.* 1983 Dec. 64(12):57, 60.

Home Health Care

Hayslip, B., and others. Home care services and the rural elderly. *Gerontologist.* 1980 Apr. 20:192-99.

Home health care for the rural elderly: experiences in Florida and Kentucky. *Pride Institute Journal of Long Term Home Health Care.* 1982 Fall. 1(2):12-19.

Kjenaas, M. A. A program to improve aftercare in a rural area. *Hospital and Community Psychiatry.* 1980 June. 31(6):401-403.

Rodell, D. E., and Jameson, J. H. Similarities and differences between an urban and a rural hospital based home care program. *Home Health Care Services Quarterly.* 1981 Winter. 2(4):29-37.

Tulga, G., and Rohrer, H. H. Developing home health care services in rural areas: a case study of decision points. *Home Health Review.* 1980 Dec. 3(4):5-11.

Hospice Care

Byrne, C. M. An assessment of the need for hospice services in a rural area. *Journal of Community Health Nursing.* 1984. 1(1):59-64.

_____. Needs assessment and hospice planning in a rural setting. *Evaluation and the Health Professions.* 1984 June. 7(2):205-19.

Jenkins, L., and Cook, A. S. The rural hospice: integrating formal and informal helping systems. *Social Work.* 1981 Sept. 26(5):414-16.

Sheehan, C. J., and Rausch, P. G. Analysis of the Medicare/hospice program: rural applicatios. *Home Health Nurse.* 1984 Sept.-Oct. 2(5):38-40.

Werner, P. T., and others. The selection and training of volunteers for a rural, home-based hospice program. *Patient Counselling and Health Education.* 1982 4th Quarter. 3(4):124-31.

Hospital Finance

Formal equipment buying plans are common, but not at small hospitals. *Modern Healthcare.* 1983 Oct. 13(10):118.

Gibson, L. E. Financing for rural hospitals. *Texas Hospitals.* 1982 Mar. 37(10):40-42.

Kolva, G. Y., Jr. Credit assistance to small hospitals. *Trustee.* 1983 May. 36(5):36.

Lightle, M. A. Capital financing tips for small hospitals. *Trustee.* 1982 Mar. 1. 35(3):38-40.

Lightle, M. A., and Hamm, M. S. Small hospitals must explore all capital options. *Hospitals.* 1980 Mar. 1. 54(5):87-90.

Patterson, A. The small hospital needs a development program. *Journal-National Association for Hospital Development.* 1983 Winter-Spring. 56-58.

Hospital Technology

Devolites, P. J. Why not high technology for the small hospital? *Computers in Healthcare.* 1984 Oct. 5(10):30-32.

Friedman, E. Small hospitals and the great technology debate. *Trustee.* 1982 Jan. 35(1):24-26.

Infection Control

Dandoy, S., and Kirkman-Liff, B. Hepatitis B prevention in small rural hospitals. *Western Journal of Medicine.* 1984 Nov. 141(5):627-30.

Bibliography

Napier, A. G. Infection control in the smaller hospital. *Texas Hospitals.* 1982 Apr. 37(11):14.

Phippen, D. E., and Williams, T. W. Manitoba's rural hospitals curtail nosocomial infections. *Dimensions in Health Service.* 1984 Sept. 61(9):26.

Scheckler, W. E. Nosocomial infection control and the smaller hospital: what do we know, what do we do? *Infection Control.* 1982 Mar.-Apr. 3(2):126.

Information Services

Brown, J. H. Telecommunications: a system for total health care. *CRC Critical Reviews in Bioengineering.* 1980. 4(4):271-309.

Cook, G. B. Clinical management by rural nurses using a microcomputer. *Journal of Medical Systems.* 1982 June. 6(3):291-94.

Garvin, J. Computers and imaging for small hospitals: present value, future growth. *Computers in Hospitals.* 1981 Nov.-Dec. 2(6):28-29.

Graham, D. L. Simultaneous remote search: a technique of providing MEDLARS services to remote locations. *Bulletin of the Medical Library Association.* 1980 Oct. 68(4):370-71.

Johnston, C. A., and Mole, A. B. Patient care computer in 68-bed hospital. *Journal of the American Medical Record Association.* 1980 Aug. 51(4):28-36.

Kabler, A. W., Reinig, E. T., and Strauch, K. P. Delivery of health-related information to rural practitioners. *Bulletin of the Medical Library Association.* 1981 Oct. 69(4):382-86.

Lochow, D., and Berger, J. D. Information and resources for rural hospitals. *Hospital Forum.* 1983 Sept.-Oct. 26(5):31-36.

Molsbee, J. A. Medium size rural hospital achieves success. *Computers in Healthcare.* 1984 Feb. 5(2):44-49.

Neely, B. One hospital's successful experience: computerization in the smaller hospital. *Texas Hospitals.* 1982 Oct. 38(5):24-26.

Swanson, S. S. Computer user groups: a shared rural hospital experience. *Healthcare Financial Management.* 1984 Nov. 38(11):76-80.

Williams, F. T., Jr. Computer applications for the smaller hospital: how to choose the right system for you. *Texas Hospitals.* 1982 Apr. 37(11):56-59.

Legislation and Health Policy

Bopp, K., and Hicks, L. State-HSA relations: state-HSA cooperation on cost containment in rural areas. *Journal of Health and Human Resources Administration.* 1981 Summer. 4(1):20-27.

Bibliography

Finch, L. E., and Christianson, J. B. Rural hospital costs: an analysis with policy implications. *Public Health Reports.* 1981 Sept.-Oct. 96(5):423-33.

Hochban, J., Ellenborgen, B., and others. The Hill-Burton program and changes in health services delivery. *Inquiry.* 1981 Spring. 18(1):61-69.

Lefton, D. Rural hospitals form new lobbying group. *American Medical News.* 1981 Oct. 16. 24(39):12.

Lichty, S. S., and Zuvekas, A. Rural health: policies, progress and challenges. *Urban Health.* 1980 Sept. 9(7):26-29.

Sussman, G. E., and Rhodes, L. Conflict between health policy and program implementation: administrative discretion and the rural health initiative. *Journal of Public Health Policy.* 1982 Mar. 3(1):64-75.

Management and Ownership Options

Alexander, J. A., and Lewis, B. L. Hospital contract management: a descriptive profile. *Health Services Research.* 1984 Oct. 19(4):461-77.

Benjamin, R. C. Contract management in a small hospital. *Michigan Hospitals.* 1980 Feb. 16(2):14-15.

Berger, J. D. Rural affiliations: why are large systems interested in rural hospitals? what do they offer? and what are they looking for? *Hospital Forum.* 1983 Sept.-Oct. 26(5):23-29.

DiPaolo, V. Investor-owned systems: for-profits target smaller hospitals. *Modern Healthcare.* 1980 Apr. 10(4):86-87.

Hughes, R. L. Small Utah hospital engineers successful financial turnaround. *Hospitals.* 1980 Dec. 16. 54(24):97-98, 100-102, 104 passim.

Multi-hospital systems: phenomenon of the past: wave of the future for industry. *Review-Federation of American Hospitals.* 1983 May-June. 16(3):20-29.

Paulsen, R. A. The role of the multi-hospital system in the survival of the smaller hospitals. *Texas Hospitals.* 1981 Mar. 36(10):30-33.

Punch, L. Alliances tailoring programs to meet small hospitals' needs. *Modern Healthcare.* 1984 Sept. 14(12).166.

_____. Rural tertiary hospitals join forces to compete with encroaching chains. *Modern Healthcare.* 1982 Nov. 12(11):44.

System ties boost small, rural accreditations. *Multis.* 1984 June. 2(2):6, 8.

Mental Health

Boydston, J. C. Rural mental health: a partnership with physicians. *Practice Digest.* 1983 Summer. 6(1):23-25.

Bibliography

Buck, J. A. Effects of the community mental health centers program on the growth of mental health facilities in nonmetropolitan areas. *American Journal of Community Psychology.* 1984 Oct. 12(5):609-22.

Flaskerud, J. H., and Kviz, F. J. Determining the need for mental health services in rural areas. *American Journal of Community Psychology.* 1984 Aug. 12(4):497-509.

_____. Resources rural consumers indicate they would use for mental health problems. *Community Mental Health Journal.* 1982 Summer. 18(2):107-19.

_____. Rural attitudes toward and knowledge of mental illness and treatment resources. *Hospital and Community Psychiatry.* 1983 Mar. 34(3):229-33.

Heiman, E. M. The psychiatrist in a rural CMHC. *Hospital and Community Psychiatry.* 1983 Mar. 34(3):227-29.

Ozarin, L. Mental health services in rural America. *Hospital and Community Psychiatry.* 1983 Mar. 34(3):197.

Perlman, B., and Hartman, E. A. The community health care administrator project: characteristics and problems of rural administrators. *Journal of Mental Health Administration.* 1983 Spring. 10(1):15-18.

Perls, S. R., Winslow, W. W., and Pathak, D. R. Staffing patterns in community mental health centers. *Hospital and Community Psychiatry.* 1980 Feb. 31(2):119-21.

Prindaville, G. M., Sidwell, L. H., and Milner, D. E. Integrating primary health care and mental health services: a successful rural linkage. *Public Health Reports.* 1983 Jan.-Feb. 98(1):67-72.

Weaver, J. D. Consultation and education in rural mental health: core elements of the (lean) 1980's. *Journal of Mental Health Administration.* 1984 Spring. 11(1):9-12.

Nursing

Arlton, D. The rural nursing practicum project. *Nursing Outlook.* 1984 July-Aug. 32(4):204-6.

Bennett, M. L. The rural family nurse practitioner: the quest for role-identity. *Journal of Advanced Nursing.* 1984 Mar. 9(2):145-55.

Benson, A. M., and others. A faculty learns about rural nursing. *Nursing and Health Care.* 1982 Feb. 3(2):78-82.

Bond, L., and others. Rural nursing: unique practice opportunity. *Michigan Nurse.* 1984 May-June. 57(3):4-6.

Bibliography

Browning, G., and Marino, P. Joint practice: a rural hospital can make it work. *Nursing Management.* 1983 Mar. 14(3):22-25.

Burfiend, M. K., and Bernhardt, T. Rural consortium: key resource for critical care nursing education. *Cross-Reference on Human Resources Management.* 1982 July-Aug. 12(4):1-5.

The FNS demonstration: where has it led? *Frontier Nursing Service Quarterly Bulletin.* 1984 Autumn. 60(2):25-28.

Halcomb, R. Frontier Nursing Service: a model for rural health care. *Nursing Careers.* 1982 Jan.-Feb. 3(1):12-13.

Jato, M. N., and others. Community participation in rural health care. *International Nursing Review.* 1984 Nov.-Dec. 31(6):180-81, 183.

Kviz, F. J., and others. Rural health care consumers' perceptions of the nurse practitioner role. *Journal of Community Health.* 1983 Summer. 8(4):248-62.

Lieveroff, A. J. Why practice in a small town? *Nursing Careers.* 1980 Sept. 1(2):6.

McDowell, H. M. Family nurse practitioners. *International Nursing Review.* 1984 Nov.-Dec. 31(6):177-79.

McMillin, B. A. On being a manager in rural Montana. *Nursing Management.* 1983 Aug. 14(8):34-36.

Morgan, W. A., and Sullivan, N. D. Nurse practitioner and physician's assistant clinics in rural California. Part 1, Issues. *Western Journal of Medicine.* 1980 Feb. 132(2):171-78.

Morgan, W. A. Nurse practitioner and physician's assistant clinics in rural California. Part 2, A survey. *Western Journal of Medicine.* 1980 Mar. 132(3):259-64.

Pedersen, B. A pilot project for training traditional birth attendants. *Journal of Nurse-Midwifery.* 1985 Jan.-Feb. 30(1):43-47.

Rolshoven, R. Rural nursing: a challenge—not for everyone. *Nursing Careers.* 1982 Jan.-Feb. 3(1):10.

Schrim, V. M., and others. Aspects of emergency nursing in rural areas. *Journal of Emergency Nursing.* 1981 Mar.-Apr. 7(2):44-46.

Stuart-Burchardt, S. Rural nursing. *American Journal of Nursing.* 1982 Apr. 82(4):616-18.

Stuart-Siddall, S. Backwoods nursing. *Nurse Educator.* 1981 May-June. 6(3):14-17.

_____. For rural nurses only? or nurses everywhere? *Home Healthcare Nurse.* 1984 Jan.-Feb. 2(1):6.

Thornton, J. M. Developing a rural nursing clinic. *Nurse Educator.* 1983 Summer. 8(2):24-29.

Bibliography

Nursing Homes

Pomeranz, B., and Breger, B. Facility financing for nursing homes. *Nursing Homes.* 1981 May-June. 30(3):2-6.

System's rural hospital expands community role. *Hospital Progress.* 1982 Oct. 63(10):24.

Pharmacy

Ambrose, J. M. Organizing pharmacy purchases in a small hospital. *Hospital Pharmacy.* 1980 Jan. 15(1):7-14.

Davis, N. M. Twenty-four hour pharmacy service in hospitals with less than 300 beds—part 2. *Hospital Pharmacy.* 1983 Aug. 18(8):421-28.

Grabowski, B. S. Staffing for comprehensive pharmaceutical services in a small hospital. *American Journal of Hospital Pharmacy.* 1981 Nov. 38(11):1708-12.

Grabowski, B. S., and Tanner, D. J. Shared Pharmaceutical services in small hospitals. *American Journal of Hospital Pharmacy.* 1980 Nov. 37(11):1534-36.

Oakley, R. S. Pharmacy practice in a small pediatric hospital. *American Journal of Hospital Pharmacy.* 1984 Apr. 41(4):694-97.

Soflin, D., Tilson, C., and Gourley, D. R. Comprehensive pharmacy services and their impact on nursing services in a 40-bed hospital. *Hospital Pharmacy.* 1980 Nov. 15(11):542-44, 548-55.

Physician Recruitment

De Castanos, O. SEARCH program targets rural physician shortage. *Colorado Medicine.* 1984 Dec. 81(12):313-14.

Downs, C. R. "Smalltown": a case history of physician retentionitis. *Michigan Medicine.* 1980 Dec. 79(35):653-54.

Glenn, J. K., and Hofmeister, R. W. Rural training settings and practice location decision. *Journal of Family Practice.* 1981 Sept. 13(3):377-82.

Goldsmith, S. B. Rural health personnel: management issues in availability, recruitment, and hospital relationships. *Journal of Ambulatory Care Management.* 1982 Nov. 5(4):49-63.

Hannon, S. K., and Witkin, M. B. Cooperative effort helps a small hospital recruit physicians. *Trustee.* 1983 Sept. 36(9):33-34.

Morris, R. L. Physician recruitment for a rural hospital. *Case Studies in Health Administration.* 1980. 2:216-23.

Porters, S. Wanted: a few good doctors for a lot of small towns. *Ohio State Medical Journal.* 1984 Aug. 80(8):589-91.

Prospective Pricing Systems (PPS)

Bartek, W. DRG strategies in the smaller hospital. *Texas Hospitals.* 1984 July. 40(2):16-17.

Ohrt, D. K. Observations on DRGs and rural referral hospitals. *Hospital Medical Staff.* 1984 May. 13(5):20-24.

Peterson, R. N., and Adams, C. M. CA District Court enjoins PPS implementation at rural hospital. *Health Law Vigil.* 1984 Aug. 17. 7(17):1-5.

Rural health and Medicaid. *Ohio State Medical Journal.* 1984 Feb. 80(2):118-21.

Purchasing

Buying for the small hospital, part 1. *Hospital Purchasing Management.* 1980 Feb. 5(2):5-7.

Campbell, S. Materials management in the small hospital. *Hospital Purchasing Management.* 1980 Apr. 5(4):15-16.

How effective are small-hospital PAs? *Hospital Purchasing Management.* 1981 Mar. 6(3):3-6.

Morgan, R. J., and Oswald, J. 70-bed hospital cuts forms down to size. *Purchasing Administration.* 1981 Jan. 5(1):31.

Richardson, J. C. Purchasing for the small hospital. *Hospital Material Management Quarterly.* 1981 May. 2(4):45-48.

Steele, R. A. Purchasing/inventory control: new system successful for small hospital. *Hospital Purchasing Management.* 1983 Jan. 8(1):14.

VanDerLinde, L. P. System to maximize inventory performance in a small hospital. *American Journal of Hospital Pharmacy.* 1983 Jan. 40(1):70-73.

Quality Assurance

Bartek, W. Developing the smaller hospital's QA program. *Texas Hospitals.* 1982 Apr. 37(11):9-10.

Davis, S., and Bryant, J. Quality assurance for the small hospital. *Times.* 1980 Nov. 21(8):4-5.

Bibliography

Langenfeld, M. L., and Rzasa, C. B. A model for integrating the quality assurance activities of two small hospitals. *Quality Review Bulletin.* 1981 Oct. 7(10):32-36.

Marsh, L. A. Quality assurance activities in a small community hospital. *QRB. Quality Review Bulletin.* 1983 Mar. 9(3):77-80.

Moeller, D. What's so different about quality assurance in small, rural hospitals? *Hospitals.* 1981 June 1. 55(11):77.

Moore, S. L. A QA program in a small rural hospital. *Quality Review Bulletin.* 1983 Aug. 9(8):233-36.

Spencer, H. J. The small hospital administrator as Q.A. coordinator. *Hospital Topics.* 1983 Nov.-Dec. 61(6):28.

Rehabilitation

Adams, M., and Whitworth, J. W. Georgia Heart Clinic: cardiac rehab in a rural setting. *Southern Hospitals.* 1984 July-Aug. 52(4):38-40.

Cordes, D. G. Health in rural Texas: focus your attention on the Tyler County Hospital rehabilitation center. *Texas Hospitals.* 1985 May. 40(12):28-29.

Lazarus, S. S., Page, C. M., and Barcome, D. F. Rehabilitation services in rural communities: delivery by hospital based and local teams. *Archives of Physical Medicine and Rehabilitation.* 1984 July. 65(7):383-87.

Wisley, L. D. Physical therapy services in rural hospital settings. *Physical Therapy.* 1981 Aug. 61(8):1173-74.

Social Services

Hayes, R. C. Community social work in a rural state. *Health and Social Work.* 1980 Nov. 5(4):64-71.

Plumlee, T. Providing social services in the rural community. *Texas Hospitals.* 1981 Feb. 36(9):24-25.

Wenston, S. R. Social work consultation for small hospitals. *Social Work in Health Care.* 1982 Fall. 8(1):15-26.

Strategic Planning and Marketing

Bridel, C. L., and Goldberg, D. M. Marketing strategies in rural areas. *Journal of Ambulatory Care Management.* 1981 Nov. 4(4):15-29.

David and Goliath: small hospitals take on big competition. *Profiles in Hospital Marketing.* 1984 2nd Quarter. 14:62-69.

Bibliography

Evans, N. E. AWHERF pioneers a rural alliance: year one. *Hospital Forum.* 1983 Sept.-Oct. 26(5):15-17, 20-21.

Fortney, D. Survival strategies for rural health care. *Hospital Medical Staff.* 1980 June. 9(6):32-37.

Frymier, B. *Productivity Improvement Is the Major Goal of This Small Hospital's Long-Range Plan.* Chicago: American Hospital Association, Center for Hospital Management Engineering, 1980.

_____. Small rural hospitals cope with the '80s. *Health Services Manager.* 1982 June. 15(6):11-13.

_____. 10-year plan lowers unused bed capacity of small rural hospital. *Hospitals.* 1981 Sept. 1. 55(17):56-57.

Gillikin, P., Price, L., and others. A self-supporting library service in a rural region: a new look at hospital consortia. *Bulletin of the Medical Library Association.* 1982 Apr. 7(2):216-23.

Hague, J. E., Harenski, R. J., and Schweighardt, G. The little hospital that could. *Hospitals.* 1980 May 16. 54(10):104-7.

Hospital adopts competitive long-range growth plan. *Hospitals.* 1982 Apr. 16. 56(8):63-64, 66.

Kelemen, J. D. Marketing and promotion: a small hospital's road to success. *Michigan Hospitals.* 1982 Mar. 18(3):27-28.

Leist, J. C. Management development imperative in small/rural hospitals. *Cross-Reference on Human Resource Management.* 1980 Sept.-Oct. 10(5):1-3.

Munroe, S. A., and Schuman, J. Small/rural hospitals must innovate in '80. *Hospitals.* 1980 Jan. 1. 54(1):99-101.

91-acre site offers design planning advantages. *Hospitals.* 1981 Mar. 16. 55(6):59-62.

Options for rural hospitals: local and regional approaches to identifying health care needs and sharing services. *Hospital Forum.* 1983 Sept.-Oct. 26(5):42-43.

Paulsen, R. A. Human touch: the smaller hospital's best medicine. *Texas Hospitals.* 1982 Apr. 37(11):54-55.

Porter-O'Grady, T., and Harrell, R. D. Transitional management: planned change in a rural hospital. *Health Care Management Review.* 1980 Summer. 5(3):39-51.

Punch, L. Alliances tailoring programs to meet small hospitals' needs. *Modern Healthcare.* 1984 Sept. 14(12):166.

_____. Rural for-profits make small profits. *Modern Healthcare.* 1983 June. 13(6):46.

Bibliography

———. Rural, tertiary hospitals join forces to compete with encroaching chains. *Modern Healthcare.* 1982 Nov. 12(11):44.

Rabinowitz, M. J., and O'Keefe, J. J., III. A prescription for ailing rural hospitals. *Trustee.* 1981 June. 34(6):45.

Reilly, B. J., and Legge, J.S., Jr. Saving the rural community hospital: an endangered species. *Hospital and Health Services Administration.* 1980. 25(Special Issue 2):17-23.

Ross, D. E. Planning for survival in small and rural hospitals. *Hospitals.* 1980 June 16. 54(12):65-70.

Rowley, B. D., and Baldwin, D. C., Jr. Assessing rural community resources for health care: the use of health services catchment area economic marketing studies. *Social Science and Medicine.* 1984. 18(6):525-29.

System's rural hospital expands community role. *Hospital Progress.* 1982 Oct. 63(10):24.

Weckworth, V. E. Small, rural hospitals: an exciting future is possible. *Michigan Hospitals.* 1980 Feb. 16(2):4-6.

Zuckerman, S. L., Dachelet, C. Z., and Westerman, J. H. Rural hospitals obtain services in 'cooperative.' *Hospitals.* 1980 May 1. 54(9):121-22, 124.

Swing Beds

Burton, R. D. Swing-bed concept in Utah: a decade of experience 1982. *Journal of Patient Account Management.* 1982 Apr.-May. 10-16.

Hanus, J. Two rural hospitals' projects apply swing bed concept successfully. *Hospital Progress.* 1980 May. 61(5):63-65.

Jessee, W. F. Quality assurance: evaluating services of small, swing-bed hospitals. *Hospitals.* 1982 Nov. 56(22):74-77.

Leaver, W. The swing bed concept. *Michigan Hospitals.* 1980 Feb. 16(2):20-22.

Pennell, F. Reimbursement: 'carve-out' method benefits swing-bed hospitals. *Hospitals.* 1982 Nov. 16. 56(22):79-80.

Shannon, K. Swing-bed program's success spurs proposals to expand eligibility. *Hospitals.* 1985 March 1. 59(5):78.

Shaughnessy, P. W., Breed, L. D., and Landes, D. P. Assessing the quality of care provided in rural swing bed hospitals. *Quality Review Bulletin.* 1982 May. 8(5):12-20.

Shaughnessy, P. W., and Schlenker, R. E. Planning: implementing new swing-bed programs. *Hospitals.* 1982 Nov. 16. 56(22):86-90.

Bibliography

Supplitt, J. T., ed. *A Swing-Bed Planning Guide for Rural Hospitals.* Chicago: American Hospital Publishing, Inc., 1984.

Supplitt, J. T. Swing beds: new diversification opportunity for small and rural hospitals. *Hospitals.* 1982 Nov. 16. 56(22):67-68.

Swing bed concept may solve rural dilemmas. *Hospital Peer Review.* 1982 Apr. 7(4):47-48.

Swing-beds meet patients needs and improve hospitals' cash-flow. *Hospitals.* 1982 July 1. 56(13):39-40.

Walter, B. A., West, J. D., and Elggren, M. D. Small hospitals find swing beds profitable. *Forum.* 1980 June. 4(2):16-17.

American Hospital Publishing, Inc.
211 East Chicago Avenue
Chicago, Illinois 60611